HOW TO SURVIVE YOUR

NURSING OR MIDWIFERY COURSE

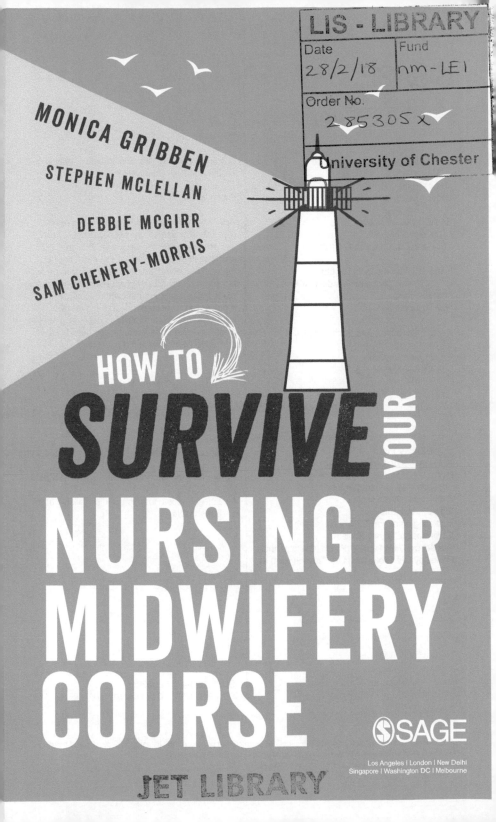

MONICA GRIBBEN
STEPHEN MCLELLAN
DEBBIE MCGIRR
SAM CHENERY-MORRIS

HOW TO
SURVIVE YOUR
NURSING OR
MIDWIFERY
COURSE

SAGE

Los Angeles I London I New Delhi
Singapore I Washington DC I Melbourne

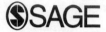

Los Angeles | London | New Delhi
Singapore | Washington DC | Melbourne

SAGE Publications Ltd
1 Oliver's Yard
55 City Road
London EC1Y 1SP

SAGE Publications Inc.
2455 Teller Road
Thousand Oaks, California 91320

SAGE Publications India Pvt Ltd
B 1/I 1 Mohan Cooperative Industrial Area
Mathura Road
New Delhi 110 044

SAGE Publications Asia-Pacific Pte Ltd
3 Church Street
#10-04 Samsung Hub
Singapore 049483

© Monica Gribben, Stephen McLellan, Debbie McGirr and Sam Chenery-Morris 2017

First published 2017

Editor: Becky Taylor
Assistant editor: Charlène Burin
Production editor: Katie Forsythe
Copyeditor: Rosemary Campbell
Proofreader: Philippu May
Indexer: Gary Kirby
Marketing manager: Tamara Navaratnam
Cover design: Wendy Scott
Typeset by: C&M Digitals (P) Ltd, Chennai, India
Printed by CPI Group (UK) Ltd, Croydon, CR0 4YY

Library of Congress Control Number: 2016946429

British Library Cataloguing in Publication data

A catalogue record for this book is available from the British Library

ISBN 978-1-4739-6922-3
ISBN 978-1-4739-6923-0 (pbk)

CONTENTS

Making and taking notes 113

Continuous assessment 117

Making it all add up – numeracy and drug calculations 129

Practical clinical skills 133

Practice learning placement 134

Making the most of your university and practice learning placement feedback 136

7 Reflective practice 139

Reflective practice – what is it exactly? 140

In-action, on-action reflection – what's the difference? 142

The ELG process 145

3Rs – recap, review, reflect 150

The reflective practitioner – continuing professional development 153

8 Making theory make sense in clinical practice 156

Taught theory and practice realities – making it all make sense 157

Transferable skills – student to practitioner, clinic to clinic 160

5Rs – recap, review, reflect, revisit, refresh 162

9 Fitness to practise – how to be a safe and professional nurse or midwife 169

Social media and your 'online self' 170

Duty of care, advocacy and whistleblowing 172

Safeguarding and protecting vulnerable groups 176

Patient safety and infection control 177

LIST OF FIGURES

ABOUT THE AUTHORS

Monica Gribben (editor) is a dyslexia specialist with a background in languages and education. She works as Dyslexia Adviser at Edinburgh Napier University and, in a private capacity, as Dyslexia Consultant to corporate organisations.

Monica has widespread experience in student support, specialising in Scottish and Norwegian University support systems for students with dyslexia. Throughout her career, she has worked extensively with student nurses and midwives.

Monica currently sits on the Scottish Government's Working Party Group on Dyslexia and is author of *The Study Skills Toolkit for Students with Dyslexia.*

Debbie McGirr (author) is a Child Health Nursing Lecturer at Edinburgh Napier University with an extended role as School Disability Contact, responsible for supporting students with additional learning needs. Debbie is qualified in Adult, Child and District Nursing, and has a wide range of experience in Community Children's Nursing.

Debbie is currently Lead Clinician with CEN – the NHS Scotland, National Managed Clinical Network for Children with Exceptional Healthcare Needs. Debbie has also contributed to edited works on healthcare-related issues.

Stephen McLellan (author) is a Careers Adviser at Edinburgh Napier University and Secretary of the University's UNISON Branch. Throughout his career, Stephen has worked extensively with student nurses and midwives.

Sam Chenery-Morris (author) is an Associate Professor, lecturing in Midwifery at the University of Suffolk. She also sits on the Faculty's Ethics Committee.

Sam is qualified in Child Health Nursing, Adult Nursing and Midwifery, working as a practitioner in these areas. She has authored, co-authored and contributed to many works in healthcare-related issues. Sam's PhD research on grading student midwives' practice is due for submission in 2016.

ACKNOWLEDGEMENTS

We've encouraged and supported each other from the first word on the first page to the final word on the last, but we've not been alone in that process. There were others who did the same and so we'd like to say 'thank you'.

Firstly, our deepest gratitude goes to Becky Taylor, Editor, for inviting us to take on this work and for her support, and to Charlène Burin, Assistant Editor, for 'keeping us right' and supporting us throughout the project. Thanks also to Katie Forsythe, Production Editor, for overseeing the production process, and to all at SAGE involved in making this idea become a reality!

Coming from two different areas in higher education – student support and nursing and midwifery teaching – meant that we didn't 'know it all', and so had to call upon the wisdom of others to ensure the information and advice we're giving you reflects the latest changes (and, of course, things may still change!).

'Thank you' to Letitia Friary, Funding Manager, Edinburgh Napier University, for keeping us right on the funding issues in Chapter 2 of this handbook – again subject to change! We're grateful to the reviewers for their comments and advice, and to Fran, Randi, Sharon, Morag, Jonathan and Laura for their comments and encouragement; we took everything on board and hope we 'got it right', doing justice to the book and the nursing and midwifery professions.

Chapter 3 on communication suggests all healthcare staff introduce themselves with 'Hello, My name is...' This introduction was inspired by Dr Kate Granger when she was having treatment for cancer.

Unfortunately, on 23 July 2016 Kate died. Not only did she spearhead the campaign, she raised thousands of pounds for charity and wrote books on her battle with cancer. She was an inspiration.

Finally, we're grateful to our artists – Gerry McGirr (Debbie's husband) for our ABC Cards, Purse, and Thermometer sketches, to Lewis Thomas Stevenson (Monica's nephew) for his student support first aider heart-valve design idea for use in Chapter 2, and to Jonathan Ryan Stevenson (Monica's nephew) for permission to use his Note Nugget sketch from *The Study Skills Toolkit for Students with Dyslexia* (2012).

PUBLISHER'S ACKNOWLEDGEMENTS

The Publishers would also like to thank David Woodroffe for his work on the illustrations and the following lecturers for their invaluable feedback on the proposal and draft chapters:

Gail Anderson, Queen's University Belfast, UK

Kim Eaton, University of Wolverhampton, UK

Claire McGuinness, Glasgow Caledonian University, UK

Amanda Smith, University of Southampton, UK

As well as the following students and newly qualified practitioners for their helpful comments on the draft material:

Sharon Patterson, Former Student Nurse At Napier University Edinburgh, UK

Melissa Cohen, Karen Henry, and Sasha Taylor, all Midwifery students at University Campus Suffolk, UK

HOW TO USE THIS HANDBOOK
READ ME, I'M IMPORTANT!

So you want to be a nurse or a midwife then? That's it, decision made! But as you take your first steps through the university doors we have to ask – do you realise your life is about to change forever, starting right now? Never thought about that, did you? Well, fortunately we did! And to help you enjoy your time at university and fully understand this change and all its challenges so you stick with the programme, we've written this handbook just for you. Answering questions you don't even know you've yet to ask, this reference tool should help you to:

- realise you're not alone on this professional journey
- gain some perspective on the demands of following a nursing or midwifery programme
- understand your assignments and achieve your learning outcomes
- make the connection between classroom theory and practice learning placements
- know what it means to maintain professional standards, from basic communication to professional conduct and competencies
- acquire insight into the legal and ethical responsibilities and expectations of being a nurse or a midwife
- learn about support networks and how they work, so when you identify your own support needs you can quickly tap into what's available, exactly when you need it most

- explore and shape your career and speciality choices, and see your continuous professional development provide new opportunities in your nursing or midwifery life, once you're qualified and registered
- discover new tools and strategies from our nursing and midwifery toolkit at the end of the book. This toolkit is packed full of visual, auditory and tactile aids to suit your own way of working and learning; use it to devise your own personalised toolkit
- take on board our top tips to help make juggling study, placement and family life work for you.

So, in this book we touch on many different topics, giving you lots of information about all the various 'bits and pieces' that make up your story as a nurse or a midwife. But what's the best way to make the most of this handbook so it all works for you? Easy! It's a handbook, so there's no need to read it from cover to cover – that approach just won't work. Read it by simply dipping in and out of the different chapters as and when you need them, and follow the story as it unfolds on a path that's specific to you in your professional journey.

The 'at a glance' content outline of each chapter should make dipping in and out easier as it points you to the information you need to read up on, exactly when you need it most. The varied visual, auditory and tactile activities should help you to identify your own learning style and develop strategies that work best for you in both your learning and your practice. But we didn't want to leave it there, so we developed a Nursing and Midwifery Toolkit packed with visual, auditory and tactile tools to help support you through the programme. And, of course, there's the friendly language style we use to make our explanations and your understanding feel less stuffy and more accessible and manageable, in your aim of becoming a safe and professional practitioner. So mix and match what's on offer, and stick with the programme!

A word of caution though when it comes to writing academic assignments. Different universities, programmes, modules and lecturers have different preferences for writing and referencing styles in different academic assignments, so always check with them the style they'd prefer you to use, and follow this advice closely. Whatever you do, don't write your academic assignments using the friendly, conversational style we're using in this handbook – chatty jargon, contractions (you'll, don't) or starting sentences with conjunctions (and, but) – it just won't work, and what's more you'll lose those valuable marks. Learn how to write academically – we've told you about that too.

Something extra to note: different universities use different terminology for people's job titles; it might be Personal Tutor in one university, Personal Development Tutor or Director of Studies in another. We've opted to use the latter two. So when it comes to the different university people, support systems and processes, check it all out so you know exactly who's who and what they're called, so you understand exactly how things work, and how it should all work for you.

So keep the goal in mind, remember to refer to your handbook often, don't be afraid to ask when you don't know or understand, remember to tap into the support available when you need it most, and, above all, believe in your own ability to stick with it and achieve that goal. Little steps, small challenges, big changes and even bigger rewards – enjoy!

1

SO YOU WANT TO BE A NURSE OR A MIDWIFE?

⇒ Stepping out into university as a nursing or midwifery student
⇒ Nursing and Midwifery Council Standards and Competencies and Professional Code
⇒ Managing expectations – academically and professionally
⇒ Professional qualities, values, principles and assumptions
⇒ Balancing academic studies, practice learning placements and family life
⇒ Practice learning placements – unlocking the fear of your first one
⇒ Writing academic assignments
⇒ Managing emotions in a caring profession

🔭 CHAPTER OVERVIEW

This chapter introduces you to the fundamentals of choosing nursing or midwifery as a profession, helping you to manage both the academic and professional elements of your education. It highlights the Nursing and Midwifery Council (NMC) standards for pre-registration midwifery education (2009) and nursing education (NMC 2010), standards for competence for registered nurses (NMC 2014) and the rules and standards for midwives (NMC 2012), so that the core principles and values of nursing and midwifery become an integral part of your development, and enable you to achieve the required standards in becoming a confident, competent and compassionate professional. To ensure you achieve both in university and in your practice learning placement, this chapter also introduces you to the three key tools you'll need to

(Continued)

(Continued)

understand and apply from the outset – your learning style, academic writing style, and time management.

- Stepping out into university as a nursing or midwifery student
- Nursing and Midwifery Council Standards and Competencies and Professional Code
- Managing expectations – academically and professionally
- Professional qualities, values, principles and assumptions
- Balancing academic studies, practice learning placements and family life

  o Finding your learning style, finding your rhythm
  o Time management – juggling, struggling or actually managing
  o So what's it to be – juggling, struggling or managing?

- Practice learning placements – unlocking the fear of your first one

  o Cementing your mentor relationship

- Writing academic assignments
- Managing emotions in a caring profession
- Top tips

STEPPING OUT INTO UNIVERSITY AS A NURSING OR MIDWIFERY STUDENT

So you've gone and done it! You've consciously taken that first step through the university doors to start your nursing or midwifery programme. Excited, scared or a bit of both? You've thought about this a great deal and you've prepared as best you can, and the way you see it this day has been a long time coming and you can't wait to get started. There's a great buzz around the university – meeting new people, where's the lecture hall, oh, there's the library, grab a quick coffee, check out the computing hub – and it seems like everybody's in the same boat. Or are they? Sure your goal is the same – pass everything, get a good degree and land that job, but...

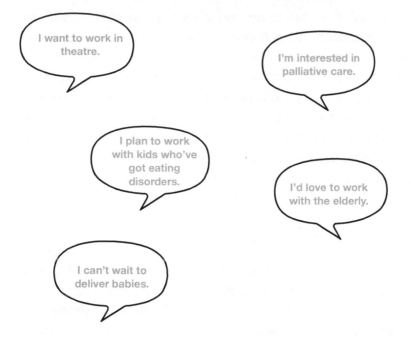

Great! You've all an Idea of what you want to do then. So first things first – what brought you here? What key qualities can you offer to this profession and how can you use them in your studies and practice learning placement?

ACTIVITY 1.1 PROFESSIONAL DOMAINS, PERSONAL QUALITIES – ADVERTISE YOURSELF

Go on tell me – advertise yourself, promote your uniqueness, but please, keep it real!

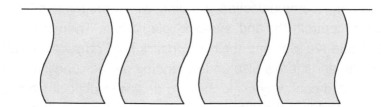

Figure 1.1 Professional domains, personal qualities – advertise yourself

So that's you! Now this is us and what we can offer – and yes, we'll keep it real too. Nursing and midwifery are great professions – personally satisfying and extremely rewarding. But step out into this programme and your life will change forever. It's extremely demanding and is a programme unlike any other at university; 50 per cent learning the theory at university and 50 per cent putting what you've learned into practice on clinical placement over your three to four year programme. In your practice learning placements, you'll work day shifts, night shifts, weekends too, while trying to keep up with university assignments and juggling everything else in your life. Early starts, late finishes, long days! So are you ready for all this?

Okay here it is – evidence-based learning, case-based learning, problem-based learning, inter-professional education, lectures, tutorials, seminars, workshops, clinical skills simulated environments, online learning materials and resources, practice placement learning. Oh, and don't forget the self-directed learning. Then there's the assessment of all that – timed written exams, short answer questions, online modules, drug calculations, multiple choice questions, reflective journals, ongoing achievement records, case studies, learning logs, oral presentations, objective structured clinical assessments (OSCAs), objective structured clinical examinations (OSCEs), essays, reports, blogs, wikis, posters, a dissertation.

And so back to you – there's your self-directed study (O'Shea 2003), matching up the reality of what happens in practice with what you've learned in the classroom, adding new knowledge to what you already know, learning new skills like critical thinking, critiquing, reflection, academic writing, note-taking, referencing, researching, communication, dealing with emotions, advocacy, infection control, oh, and avoiding plagiarism. Then there's the NMC Code (2015a) and their *Standards for Competence* (2014) to uphold, and there's also understanding professionalism – what you can and can't say or do, how to deal with difficult situations, how to report unprofessional behaviours, and how to keep yourself safe as a professional. Add to that - learning who's who and what they do in your university, sorting out your support needs, accessing what you need exactly when you need it. Phew! It reads like an encyclopaedia, I know, but just think of the end result – supported studies, personal support, your career taking shape, entry to a lifelong profession, worldwide and endless opportunities, a rewarding life.

Well, is it everything you expected when you signed up to the nursing or midwifery profession? Are you ready to take it all on board? You are! Then it's over to you now. You've stepped out into university; we'll give you the tools to manage it all. Take responsibility, keep your finger on the pulse and you'll surely stay 'on course'!

NURSING AND MIDWIFERY COUNCIL STANDARDS AND COMPETENCIES AND PROFESSIONAL CODE

Rules, regulations, professional expectations – we can't avoid them. All institutions have them and all professional bodies are enshrined in them, and the NMC is no exception. So what exactly is the NMC?

Well, it's a professional body whose main aim is to protect both patients and the public by monitoring the personal and professional activity of nurses and midwives working in the United Kingdom (UK), whether in the National Health Service (NHS) or private settings. It also protects nurses and midwives by setting standards and providing guidance on all aspects of practice. So how about some key NMC facts:

- It's directly accountable to the UK Parliament.
- It's governed by an independent council.
- It maintains a register of all registered nurses and midwives who've completed their initial training, met and continued to uphold the registration standards, and so are eligible to practise.
- It sets out a code of conduct, which all nurses and midwives must adhere to throughout their professional career, regardless of the setting – NHS or private healthcare, hospitals, the community, prisons, social care, education.

- It sets standards for pre-registration nursing and midwifery education, and supports learning and assessment of students in practice.
- It investigates and acts upon any concerns about a nurse's or midwife's conduct or actions.

So what does this mean for you – the student nurse or midwife? After all, it's your professional body too!

Well, as soon as you sign up for a student nursing or midwifery programme, you're automatically bound by the NMC Code (2015a) and its standards. From your first student placement, you'll be in the privileged position of caring for people from all walks of life, cultural backgrounds and ages, and so you're expected to act professionally, with honesty, integrity, respect and confidentiality at all times. A tall order, we know! But to manage all this, you're given guidelines that support and protect you, your patients and the staff you're working with. So what are these guidelines?

The Code (NMC 2015a) sets out four key domains (Figure 1.2), within which all nurses and midwives need to achieve the following outcomes:

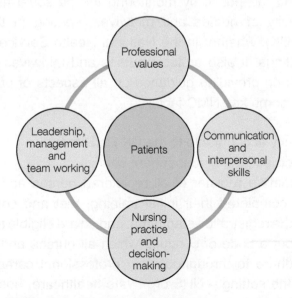

Figure 1.2   NMC four domains

Within these four key domains, you'll find knowledge, skills and values that all nurses and midwives need to meet to achieve specific levels of competence. As a student nurse or midwife, you too are expected to achieve specific competencies in practice from day one of your programme of study.

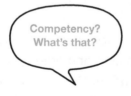

Competency? What's that?

Well, it's a way of demonstrating that you've achieved a specific level of knowledge and understanding that enables you to practise safely as a nurse or midwife. Exactly that! Without this, you can't be registered to practise. So reflect – how can you place this principle at the heart of your professional values, not only in your formative years in nursing or midwifery but in your professional role as a clinical practitioner? Have you considered too how all this might affect your personal life and how different things will be from now on?

MANAGING EXPECTATIONS – ACADEMICALLY AND PROFESSIONALLY

Being a nursing or midwifery student is all about 'managing': writing assignments, meeting deadlines, connecting theory with practice, achieving practice placement learning outcomes, adhering to The Code (NMC 2015a) professional guidelines and managing your professionalism. In short, meeting and managing academic and professional expectations from day one of university. Surprised? Yes, even at university you're expected to manage your behaviour, attitude and approach to things, not to mention respect the university's rules and regulations, as outlined in your university's Student Charter. Be mindful also of the professional expectations in your NMC Placement Charter. Building trust, confidence and respect is a 'two-way street' – our expectations are reasonable, make sure yours are too!

You expect us to inspire your learning through our teaching, support your learning in your practice learning placement, respond to your needs – academic, personal and professional – in a timely manner, and generally deliver a good service. That's our end of the bargain, now what's yours?

In return, we expect you to:

- take responsibility for your own learning and self-directed study
- adopt good organisation and time management strategies
- touch base with Student Services to arrange your initial support needs and tap into their support network when things get difficult
- engage with your university's Student Learning Environment, such as Moodle
- become familiar with the library, its search engines and borrowing processes
- make regular contact with your Personal Development Tutor/ Director of Studies (PDT/DoS)
- utilise your natural learning style effectively
- learn academic writing and use key study tools, for example, Turnitin (www.turnitinuk.com); Harvard referencing style (https:// libweb.anglia.ac.uk/referencing/harvard.htm); APA referencing style (www.ukessays.com)
- meet assignment deadlines
- make the most of feedback to help improve your written work and enhance your practice
- plan your placement journey and arrive on time
- tell us of any concerns you have about your studies, placement or personal life
- behave responsibly – after all, you're effectively an ambassador for your university and your chosen profession
- uphold the NMC Code (2015a) and its professional domains, respect the patient, their needs and rights, privacy and confidentiality
- familiarise yourself with the relevant legislative policies (Appendix 1).

Learn these skills, identify their transferable value across all health-care settings and in all your communications, and you'll surely manage as a student and develop as a confident professional.

PROFESSIONAL QUALITIES, VALUES, PRINCIPLES AND ASSUMPTIONS

The practice of nursing and midwifery is based upon values, professional principles, morals, ethics – while we'll talk more about these in Chapter 10, it's important to acknowledge their importance at the very outset of your student journey. Nursing and Midwifery are 'values-based professions' (NMC 2015a). So what does all that mean really?

Well, values are the things we hold dear – they're based on our beliefs, thoughts, knowledge and feelings, and so are important in our lives. They define us as individuals. But how do we relate all this to our nursing and midwifery practice, and what do we mean by professional qualities, attitudes, morals, ethics, values and principles? Why is it important to consider them from our very first day at university?

Well, it's all about making sure the people we're caring for are given the best possible care and choices to improve their health and well-being. It's also about working within a moral and ethical code which safeguards patients and families. These are the fundamental principles of nursing and midwifery practice and, of course, the main reason why we consciously took that first step. Don't be mistaken – applying the values we hold dear is a tall order, especially when patients' attitudes and expectations, stressful and busy working environments, and teamwork are all in the mix, and can influence our thoughts and behaviour. But we've all been patients at one time or another, and being treated with dignity, care and compassion helps our recovery. So to ensure you too can achieve this, you'll need to understand and accept the principles of the professional practice you've signed up to – be caring, non-judgemental, supportive, respectful of individuality, organised and professional at all times – no more, no less! It's these aspects of behaviour and personality that are sought after even before you get a place at university, through a values-based selection and recruitment process which helps universities to attract and employ the right people who can demonstrate and develop these key attributes (www.nmc.org.uk/; www.rcn.org.uk/; www.rcm.org.uk/). Take all this with you into your practice and you'll surely become the nurse or midwife you set out to be.

BALANCING ACADEMIC STUDIES, PRACTICE LEARNING PLACEMENTS AND FAMILY LIFE

Let's face it, we've been dragged into the 21st century with all its busyness, and despite our longing for a quiet life, we never seem to get it; we only get busier. If it's not this or that, then it's that or this; always something grabbing our attention and demanding our time – just got to keep up with what's new!

So what's new in your life now that you've started to study? Can you honestly keep up with that 5-hour lecture day, school run, after school club, dinner, homework, housework, shopping, part-time job, library search, note-taking, writing up until 1am, grabbing a few hours' sleep, early shift again at 7am, first placement. Phew! Exhausted, stressed just thinking about it? In a sentence, how do we strike the balance between our academic studies, our practice learning placement and our family life?

I suppose you've heard it said that there's a time for everything. It's true, but how we organise and utilise that time while working our way through a highly intensive programme is key to keeping on track and well. First things first though – find your learning style (http://vark-learn.com/the-vark-questionnaire/; www.businessballs. com/freepdfmaterials/vak_learning_styles_questionnaire.pdf; Honey and Mumford 2001) and your study rhythm, and you should strike a balance to a manageable, stress-free academic and professional life.

FINDING YOUR LEARNING STYLE, FINDING YOUR RHYTHM

You do it your way, I do it my way, we all do it differently – and still we learn; learn the same things, but differently. We complete our assignments and we sit our exams, and somehow we pass. For many of us, our early experience of learning was in a small class at school with follow-up homework, but will the same learning style help us learn and understand in the same way now, when lectures, practice learning placements and self-directed study are our main sources of learning? Will this learning style help us understand why we learn the way we do from these three sources? So why do we learn this way and not that?

I've only just completed my Access to Nursing course; thought my dyslexia and ADHD would've gotten in the way. I mean I know how I like to study and feel it works – quiet space free from distractions, soft background music, scribbling pad beside me so I can storyboard my ideas – hmm, not so sure now. Got this far though, but still trying to figure out how I really learn best.

I've come straight from school and was hopeless at knowing how to study; never could get to grips with it or understand how you're meant to study really.

Okay, so we need to make sure your learning style works well for you so that you:

- understand lectures and how they work
- know how to get the most from your practice learning placements
- get to grips with self-directed study.

And overall, we need make sure you can make the connections between all three learning sources and understand what you need to learn and why. So what kind of learner are you?

⚓ ACTIVITY 1.2   LEARNING STYLE TASK

Choose a task; tell me your story – why did you choose nursing or midwifery?

- Draw a picture = visual.
- Write a letter = auditory.
- Design and create something = tactile.

So which one did you instinctively choose? Doesn't that tell you something about your learning style? Still not sure how all this works? Then complete Activity 1.3 (see Appendix 2 for answers).

⚓ ACTIVITY 1.3   VISUAL, AUDITORY OR TACTILE LEARNER – OR SIMPLY A BIT OF EVERYTHING?

Do you:

- use mind maps or shapes to connect and understand information?
- read information aloud so you can hear it?
- record information so you can listen back?
- use colours to highlight information and then read it?
- tap your fingers on your arm when counting?
- discuss concepts with others?
- use colours to highlight information and then create a picture or object?
- follow a mind map more easily than written instructions?
- use music or mnemonics to learn information?
- move around or walk when you're reading?
- see patterns in information?
- enjoy practical tasks that help you learn?

(Gribben 2012: 6)

Put simply, if you prefer to see things in pictures so you can under-stand and study better, then you're clearly a visual learner. If you find that listening to information makes things sink in better, then you're an auditory learner. As for the tactile learner, well it's a case of actively doing, feeling, practising what you need to learn so it all makes sense. If you like to use strategies from some or all learning styles to help support your learning and understanding then quite simply, you're a little bit of everything. We all have our own unique way of working – systems, strategies, even rituals. There's no right or wrong way. Take time to refine the learning style that's unique to you, work with it, make it work for you, and you'll soon find your study rhythm, and with that lectures, practice learning placements, self-directed study and overall success should easily fall into place (El-Gilany and Abusaad 2012). Of course it doesn't stop there; this brings me nicely to our next point – time management. Find your study rhythm and add a good dose of time management, and your days will be more organ-ised and balanced, with more juggle and less struggle.

TIME MANAGEMENT - JUGGLING, STRUGGLING OR ACTUALLY MANAGING

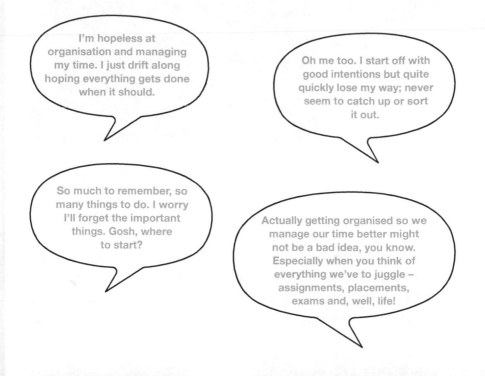

SO WHAT'S IT TO BE – JUGGLING, STRUGGLING OR MANAGING?

We arrive at university and before long we can all sometimes feel overwhelmed – by the new environment, a new life, lots of new things going on at the same time and seemingly endless pieces of information. Sometimes it feels all too much and before long we can feel things slipping and we struggle. It's not meant to be like this, I hear you say. I'm sure you've been in a similar situation before when you struggled. Correct? Then let's look at how you managed that situation and what worked for you.

ACTIVITY 1.4   MANAGING STRATEGIES – ANYTHING YOU'D DO DIFFERENTLY

What strategies have you successfully used that could help you manage this situation? Note them in the Juggling Man.

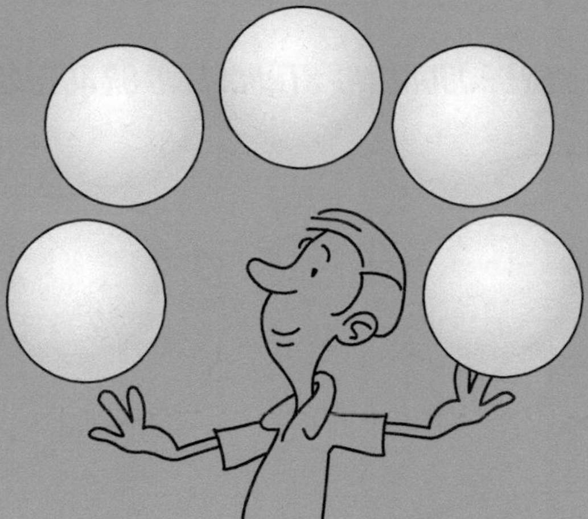

FIGURE 1.3   Juggling man

Isn't it true that when we're in the thick of the 'bad' situation it's hard to see the way ahead? We need to start somewhere, so I suppose making a timetable of your university commitments is as good a place as any – lectures, tutorials, seminars, personal development meetings … anything else? Next, consider when you study best – morning, afternoon, evening? Colour that slot into your timetable, dividing up the various times between research, reading and critical thinking, sorting information and finally writing up. So, for example, if you study best in the morning it makes sense to use that time for these tasks; you're more alert then! Then add in any family commitments. Remember, if you can delegate some of these duties, do it; having help makes life seem more manageable. And to make things even less of a juggle, learn to prioritise.

You've tried all these but still you're feeling the struggle? Then don't go it alone, tap into your Student Support First Aider (SSFA; Chapter 2) and get the support you need exactly when you need it, and not when things feel somewhat overwhelming. There's a wealth of support on offer, such as academic support to help you devise strategies to maximise your study time and manage your workload, and what about the personal support talking therapies to help you manage the stress? So, take action early; channel your energies into what's important at that moment rather than endlessly stressing and struggling and feeling hopelessly 'lost'.

And so to placements – create a new timetable that accommodates all your life at that time – practice learning placement, university assignments and family commitments. Note that it's placement time, so expect a different rhythm to your days; remember the shift pattern. As well as carrying on with all your other commitments, you need to factor in travel time to your placement. It's wise to do a trial run of the various travelling routes and times. Always check the travel forecast before setting out, take the shortest, most direct route and leave enough travel time so you're always on time!

Sure, we all travel to work, work different shifts and need to arrive on time, but when you're part of a team delivering patient care you need to consider others. You're about to start your shift, others are finishing. How do you feel when you're tired and desperate to get home, and you're waiting around for a latecomer? If a shift handover is rushed, potentially something important can be missed and mistakes made. Reflect on that! Of course, we can all oversleep or unexpectedly get stuck in a traffic jam behind an accident – once perhaps – but habitual latecomers aren't looked upon favourably. So make every effort to be on time, set your alarm, plan your journey and build yourself a good reputation as a reliable, trustworthy, committed professional who's a team player, takes work seriously and actually wants to be there. Do that and watch doors open to opportunities you never imagined. Do the right thing, facilitate a smooth handover, alleviate stress and start your shift on a positive note. But if the unexpected happens, call your placement mentor!

PRACTICE LEARNING PLACEMENTS – UNLOCKING THE FEAR OF YOUR FIRST ONE

Practice learning placements are wide-ranging and varied (Appendix 3); you get to put what you've already learned into real-life practice alongside a qualified nurse or midwife who'll be your mentor or guide throughout your placement, so make the most of it (RCN 2009; Whitehead 2013). Having attended university for a number of weeks now, your first practice learning placement is just around the corner. Excitement! Can't wait to get started; work with patients, learn from others – your mentor and team. Apprehensive too? Then take the fear out of your first placement by speaking to your mentor before you start, or emailing them; this is a great opportunity to introduce yourself, go over the basics as detailed in your student placement book, and to learn about your duties, responsibilities and rights in the placement (Levett-Jones and Bourgeois 2015). If the opportunity arises, do a trial run of the journey, meet with your mentor, see exactly where you'll work and arrange any extra support you might need because of your specific difficulties. However, this isn't always possible due to personal commitments or location, so don't worry about it – but *do* always make contact with your mentor before you arrive.

If you're wondering about your practice learning placement time sheets, learning log, writing up patient notes, passing on information, drug administration, patient confidentiality, then this is the time to ask. Get your questions answered and you'll have unlocked some of the fear of your first placement; watch the worries disappear!

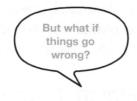

But what if things go wrong?

Sometimes, just sometimes, placements do go wrong, even for the best of us. You don't particularly connect with your mentor; it's not the interesting learning environment you thought practice would be; you're finding it all too much – placement, family life and keeping up with assignments; or the unexpected happens – personal crisis. If any of this happens, talk to your Link Lecturer or PDT/DoS, explain the situation and try to find a solution. Yes, there are solutions! Whether it's taking time out or repeating your placement, there's no shortage of support. They'll fully support you, help you to arrive at your decision and direct you to any support services you might need to use. The important thing is you don't get lost in the process, so talk to them, access the support, find a way forward; it's all there for you – yes you!

Want to avoid things going wrong? Then consider:

1. You're dealing with patient care, supporting their health and well-being, and so details about them are important. Know your role in any handover, safeguard yourself and your patient, and take time to write patient notes accurately, mindful of confidentiality (Scovell 2010). Remember, if it's important enough to say something about a patient in the handover then it's important enough to write in the notes; don't leave that important detail to memory – neither yours nor someone else's.
2. You're part of a team – arrive on time, respect individuals, communicate positively and show willing in teamwork.

3. You're still a student and still learning, so keep in touch with your university and tap into the wealth of support at your fingertips.

4. You're a student – yes, but you're bound by a code of conduct, as are your mentor and team, so if you're concerned about someone's professional practice then report it (NMC 2015b). Don't let the matter escalate into what could become a complicated or potentially serious situation.

CEMENTING YOUR MENTOR RELATIONSHIP

Relationships matter – we live, thrive and survive through our relationships with others. They encourage, support and advise us, and are often key to our success. Professional relationships are no different, except they offer something more – professional expertise. Draw on your mentor's experience so that what you learn in university makes sense in the practice learning environment. Don't forget your mentors were students too at one time – they understand you!

Of course, positive relationships with your lecturers, peers and patients are important, but the most important relationship in your formative years is with your practice learning placement mentor. Their role is to teach, support and assess you during your pre-registration period, and to sign off on your ability as 'fit to practise' and register as a nurse or midwife (RCN 2009). So take positive steps to build up trust and confidence in your relationship, respect their knowledge and experience, trust their advice and support, and be open to their feedback (Somerville and Keeling 2004; Duffy 2013). Do all this and you'll surely enjoy your practice learning placement and achieve your placement learning outcomes.

WRITING ACADEMIC ASSIGNMENTS

Writing a letter to a friend, a school magazine article or social media posts isn't quite the same as writing an academic assignment. Wouldn't student life be so much easier if it was, and we could write exactly how we speak? Language styles are very different! What's acceptable in social circles, 'text speak' or even the writing style we're using in this handbook isn't acceptable in academic assignments. Oh no! Write like this and you'll lose valuable marks.

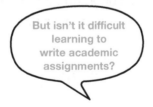

But isn't it difficult learning to write academic assignments?

No! It's just a matter of technique and rules – knowing what to write, what not to write and how, and there you have it. Remember, it's not an automatic skill; it needs to be learned and takes time! Different universities, modules and assignments use different writing styles, so always check with your tutor about the writing style they'd like you to use. Remember, too, the study skills workshops, such as 'Essay Doctor' or 'Referencing and Plagiarism', and one-to-one study support on various aspects of academic writing offered by your universities' Learning Information Services. So make finding out about all of this one of your 'Top 10' actions! After all, they're there for you! We'll cover more of this support in Chapter 2.

Writing in an academic-style language doesn't mean that you've to write in a way that's complicated, long-winded or difficult to understand. No! It has to be brief, clear, direct, straightforward, informative and readily understood by the reader. We'll cover some of the basic rules in Chapter 6. So, learn, practise and apply the academic language style early on in your studies, and you'll see how quickly it becomes part of your academic and working practice, so that you'll:

- be aware of the relevant style, its rules and its importance
- have the correct style at the forefront of your professional practice
- continually respect the appropriate writing styles as an important value in your chosen profession when producing professional emails, reports, notes and other written communications
- have no difficulty producing practice learning placement reports.

That's the writing but what about the lecturers' feedback? That's important too! So take their constructive developmental comments as a positive to help you improve and develop your future academic writing. Do all that and you'll surely gain those much needed marks, and, who knows, perhaps open doors to new professional opportunities by contributing to research papers, projects and reports.

MANAGING EMOTIONS IN A CARING PROFESSION

Nursing and Midwifery practice is personally demanding and emotionally engaging (Hunter and Deery 2009; Hunter and Warren 2013). Caring for people and facilitating well-being wherever possible is all about building and managing relationships. Managing your own emotions while dealing with others' emotional situations isn't only linked to being professional but is also required to deliver the high standard of evidence-based care laid down by your employer, and as guided by the NMC Code (2015a).

Faced with many different situations across different healthcare sectors, you'll need to build up a variety of skills to help you negotiate and deal with the varied, ever-changing demands of patients, families and peers. We're emotional beings, some more than others, but what families don't need when dealing with their own emotional situation is to deal with yours too! This doesn't mean that you should switch off your emotions – do that and you're not in the right profession! No – chat to mentors, team members, take their advice and build on that. It's all part of the learning process.

So what does this mean for you? Well, it means:

- recognising and acknowledging your own feelings in addition to those of your patients, their families, and your team members
- being able to constantly respond to changing expectations
- managing your emotions and feelings through support and supervision
- knowing how and when to disengage emotionally
- knowing how to take care of yourself.

ACTIVITY 1.5 STRENGTHS AND LIMITATIONS IN EMOTIONAL SITUATIONS

You're on your first placement and are faced with an emotional situation. How would you deal with this while also taking care of yourself? List your personal strengths and limitations, and their potential effects on the situation.

Now take a step back and reflect on your responses. Consider also your mentor's or team's advice to help you manage 'emotions' in an emotional situation? And remember, always take care of yourself – if you don't do that you'll struggle to take care of others.

So that's it – we've covered the basics of what you'll need when starting out as a student nurse or midwife. Like everything, basics are only the first layer; we'll build on this as we progress through the chapters, discussing topics more fully and providing tools to help you manage and feel supported. You've stepped out, so keep going.

TOP TIPS

✓ Read your University Student Charter, NMC Placement Charter, NMC Code, NMC Standards and Competencies, and disability legislation.

✓ In a group, discuss the professional guidelines and what they mean in your lives now.

✓ Arrange your support needs at the start of your course.

✓ Make a weekly timetable of your commitments – university, placement, family and social, and pin it on your noticeboard.

✓ Create a traffic light system of priorities so you keep on track with your studies.

✓ Create a juggling man of who's who in your university and placement.

✓ Keep a pocket size reflective diary and reflect often on your studies and your practice.

✓ Identify your natural learning style and use it effectively.

✓ Familiarise yourself with the library and its services.

(Continued)

(Continued)

✓ Practise your academic writing; create index cards of the Dos and Don'ts in academic writing, carry them with you or pin them on your noticeboard.

✓ Familiarise yourself with Turnitin.

✓ Practise the Harvard and APA referencing styles.

✓ Use storyboarding to create:

  o a glossary of medical terminology

  o graphical symbols you'd use in patient reports, e.g. draw a happy or sad face for communication, knife and fork for eating

  o a visual noting and reporting system, e.g. draw hands with symbols on them for handover of placement, use graphical associations, colours

✓ Do a trial run of the journey from your home to your placement.

✓ Manage your shifts and time-off requests using a hardcopy timetable or online ShiftHub software.

✓ Keep in touch with your university while on placement.

So those are the tips, but don't forget your toolkit at the end of the book!

FURTHER READING

Byrom, S. and Downe, S. (eds) (2015) *The Roar Behind the Silence: Why Kindness, Compassion and Respect Matter in Maternity Care*. London: Pinter & Martin Ltd.

Johnson, R. (2010) *Skills for Midwifery Practice*, 3rd edition. London: Churchill Livingstone.

Lillyman, S., Gutteridge, R. and Berridge, P. (2011) 'Using a storyboarding technique in the classroom to address end of life experiences in practice and engage student nurses in deeper reflection', *Nurse Education Practice*, 11(3): 79–86.

Medincle: www.medincle.com/

NMC (2015a) *The Code: Professional Standards of Practice and Behaviour for Nurses and Midwives*. London: NMC: www.nmc.org.uk/standards/code.

Taylor, D.B. (2012) *Writing Skills for Nursing and Midwifery Students*. London: SAGE.

The Student Room 'How to cope on nursing placements': www.thestudentroom. co.uk/wiki/how_to_cope_on_nursing_placements

2 YOU'RE MORE THAN JUST A STUDENT

→ You're more than just a student
→ Your personal situation – home, family, social
→ Your Student Support First Aider – who's who and what they do
→ Financial support
→ Academic support
→ Personal support
→ Professional support
→ Those dreaded surveys

CHAPTER OVERVIEW

Being a student is what university is all about. But with the demands of study, work, clinical placements and even family life in the mix, today's nursing and midwifery students are more than just a student. To help make juggling this 'mix' seem more manageable, this chapter gives you your Student Support First Aider (SSFA). So when the unexpected happens or the going gets tough, the key information, advice and strategies provided should help support your needs, and make your nursing and midwifery studies work well for you.

- You're more than just a student
- Your personal situation – home, family, social
- Your Student Support First Aider – who's who and what they do
- Financial support

  o Money matters
  o Full purse, empty wallet – it just doesn't add up
  o Disabled Students' Allowance – what's that?

(Continued)

(Continued)

- Academic support

  - Struggling with your studies?
  - Library
  - Information technologist
  - Keep track of your studies

- Personal support

  - Managing stressful situations
  - When the unexpected happens
  - Mitigating circumstances
  - Taking time out
  - Making your decision
  - Returning to studies
  - Disability Service
  - Health and Well-being Service
  - Coping with the emotional burden of caring

- Professional support

  - Skills, knowledge, practice – your professional questions answered

- Those dreaded surveys
- Top tips

YOU'RE MORE THAN JUST A STUDENT

Let's face it, you may have walked through the university doors to start your nursing or midwifery programme but you didn't split yourself in two and leave the other part of your life outside on the doorstep, did you? Of course you didn't; you can't! Sure you're a student, but you're also a social being with a family, part-time job, personal commitments, emotional life, worries and concerns like most of us, and life carries on. And now, well, you've signed up to this highly demanding programme that offers a new way of learning, new demands and new expectations – where every-thing changes. From day one, you need to reorganise your life, keep up with university commitments, manage your personal commitments, adapt to study-placement demands, learn all about student life, uphold the professional expectations, learn how to deal with others' emotions while dealing with your own, find answers to your many questions, and, of course, look after yourself. It's a lot to cope with, we know that. You'll have ups and downs, we know that too, and so to help you work through all this, we hope you'll feel supported with the advice and information in this chapter.

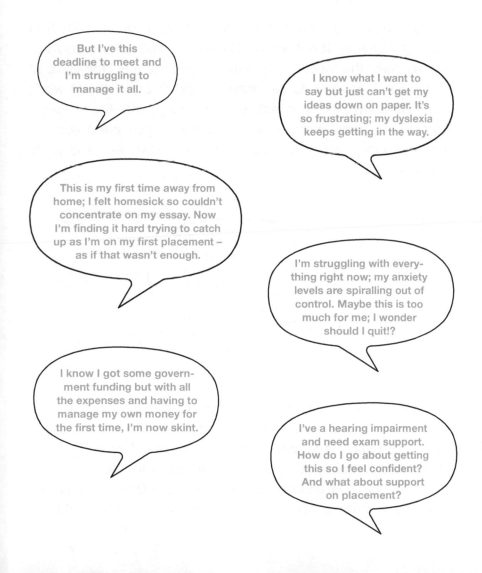

We've all been there at one time or another; we've let the small worries find a space in our head, it's hard to think of much else. That space for worrying soon gets bigger and those worries won't leave – they like it there; comfortably rolling around, sometimes even becoming firmly rooted. Stop and think! Would you rather go round and round the worry wheel or climb the progress ladder? What's that – climb? Then tackle the worry! You've heard it said – if you don't ask, you don't get; the same is true here. If you tell us you need support, you'll surely get it; if you don't then you won't – simple!

Remember, being a student is only one part of your life. Student life is short lived! Sure it's stressful but it's also fun and rewarding, so make the most of your student experience. Don't just sit on the sidelines and do the basics to get through. It just won't work! Be active, even proactive, and engage with the process. As for your small worries, if you're aware you need support then the earlier you sort it out the better – start well and you'll end well.

> But I find it hard trying to manage my family commitments alongside my university and placement commitments, and I've only just started.

Oh, that's easy to sort. Remember, you've a duty of care to look after yourself; you need to acknowledge that, so wherever you can, allocate duties to family and friends. Don't feel as if you've got to do everything yourself; you don't need to! Okay, got that sorted? Worked out duties and responsibilities? Do you feel you've achieved a more supported study-work-family-social timetable?

That's family and friends, but what about the university? What's on offer there? Well, quite a lot actually.

YOUR PERSONAL SITUATION – HOME, FAMILY, SOCIAL

We all come from families of various shapes, sizes and responsibilities. Some leave home to start university and have that longed-for independence, come and go as they please, make their own decisions and have total responsibility for their own lives, with family in the 'background'. Oh, what freedom!

Well that's you, but this is me – 38-year-old mother of four, last in education 20 years ago, partner recently made redundant, solely responsible for family chores, school run, kids' social activities – basically everything to keep family life going. Four months into my studies – work piles up, deadlines too, social life forgotten, family time scarce, 'me' time disappeared, and stress on the horizon. So tell me, how can I keep on top of my studies and make sure my home life is manageable? Easy – time management! Reflect again on your work-study-family-social timetable. Need any adjustments? Make them! Can your partner take on extra tasks? Allocate them! Managing to be a student while maintaining your personal life is all about organisation, time management (www.studymore.org.uk/timetips.htm) and those small adjustments where others step out to support you. And on the days when the going gets tough, well that's when your SSFA is on tap to help. So whether leaving home or staying home, young or mature – balancing your student and your personal life is key to success.

YOUR STUDENT SUPPORT FIRST AIDER – WHO'S WHO AND WHAT THEY DO

Oh, don't you wish everything in life was plain sailing, but it isn't like that, and we know that. Sometimes things happen and we become unstuck; we fret and worry and need a helping hand.

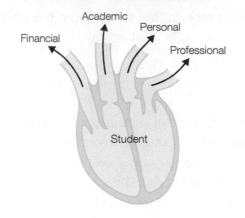

Figure 2.1   Student Support First Aider

Student life is no exception; you'll have many ups and downs. So for the many times you're feeling unstuck, we're giving you your SSFA (Figure 2.1).

Remember, whether it's multi-campus or just one, the Student Services – Hub, Enquiry Centre, One-Stop-Shop, whatever it's called – is essentially the one place in university you'll need to know about. Where can I find what's on offer? What can I access? The answer is everything you need to know at some point along the way when that little hiccup occurs in your studies and you feel stuck, unsettled, lost, maybe even desperate. So, from drop-in sessions for quick advice or guidance to appointment slots, support services does what it says on the label – 'supports'; gives you a helping hand to get back on track, becoming motivated and focused again so that 'de-stress' not 'distress' (see e.g., Mental Health in Manchester, www.mhim.org.uk/helpguides/) is key in your student life. So note the support.

ACTIVITY 2.1   NOTE THE SUPPORT

Note the key support services you'll definitely use, where you'll find them and what they offer.

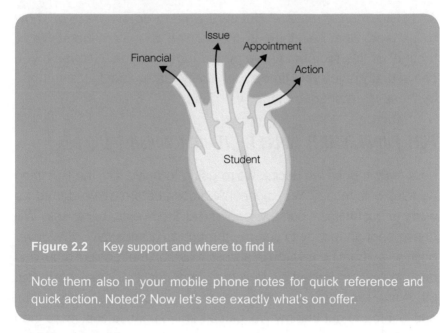

Figure 2.2   Key support and where to find it

Note them also in your mobile phone notes for quick reference and quick action. Noted? Now let's see exactly what's on offer.

FINANCIAL SUPPORT

It's in the purse and out of the wallet – everything you need to know about managing your student finances.

MONEY MATTERS

We need it; can't do without it, and yet sometimes we just don't have enough to make ends meet, and we worry. We've applied early for our fees, bursary, loan, childcare fund, disabled students' allowance (DSA) to ensure it's all in place for starting:

- www.saas.gov.uk/
- www.gov.uk/student-finance
- www.sfengland.slc.co.uk/
- www.studentfinancewales.co.uk/
- www.studentfinanceni.co.uk/
- www.hea.ie/

And still – money matters! Not sure what to do, where to go, how to manage, what help there is, if any? Yes, money matters! We've thought of this too, and we've pulled together a few ideas so you can actually enjoy your time at university rather than feel swamped by those mismanaged money worries.

FULL PURSE, EMPTY WALLET – IT JUST DOESN'T ADD UP

Let's face it, once we decide we're going to university, the first thing we think of is money. Yes, money! And even before we've started we worry about the fees, bursary, loan and all those extra expenses. 'Will I have enough money to see me through to graduation?' 'I've never been away from home before; always relied on the "bank of mum and dad" so I'm wondering how I'll actually manage it all'. Well that's you, this is me. I've single parent commitments, a home and family to run, and just found out that my first placement expenses cost more than expected. How am I supposed to manage all that? Oh, and you think that's bad – I went on a spending spree and am running out of money already. It's easy to spend too much on 'wants' instead of 'needs'.

Look we've all been there, spent our last penny on that 'must have' pair of shoes, eaten a sandwich instead of a cooked meal, mis-calculated this month's budget – ending up with an empty piggy bank! Let's be budget aware and money wise! And if you don't know how, just say – we're here to help!

But what happens if I run out of money? Even if I'm down to my last £20 I'd rather not ask; I'd feel embarrassed. You know I never realised what it all costs to live away from home, rent a flat, pay for heating and lighting, travel, buy books, food, and then there's my social life. What about my gym membership and my night out with flatmates?

Let's take a step back. You've taken that first step through the university doors because you're intent on becoming a nurse or midwife; you're committed to your studies but now you've reached a bad patch. Are you going to let poor budgeting or overspending get in the way of achieving your dream? Surely not, when all it takes is three little words – 'I need help'. Say that and we'll advise, support and even help you out of that sticky situation. Trying to be independent doesn't mean you won't need help at some point; we all do. So let's take a look at how you're spending your money just now and what's an 'I need' and an 'I want'.

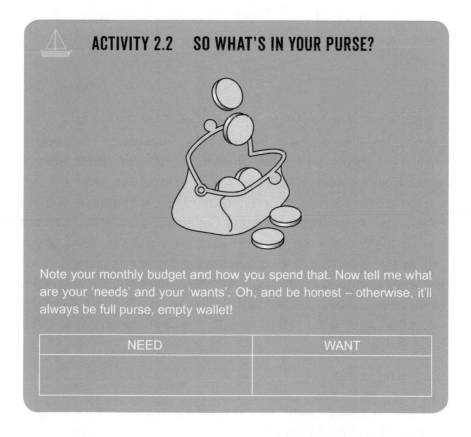

ACTIVITY 2.2   SO WHAT'S IN YOUR PURSE?

Note your monthly budget and how you spend that. Now tell me what are your 'needs' and your 'wants'. Oh, and be honest – otherwise, it'll always be full purse, empty wallet!

NEED	WANT

So what's the cost of your 'wants'? Planning to avoid money mismanagement and debt? Then check out the National Union of Students (NUS) budgeting information (www.nus.org.uk/en/advice/money-and-funding/money-budgeting-/) or talk to your university's

Funding Team to help you work out a realistic monthly budget or manage your debt. Done? Now prioritise! Forget the social night this week; pay your commitments – rent, energy bills, household expenses, car, phone, insurance. Done! Any pennies left? Pop them in your piggy bank, save for what you want and you'll value it more. That's the budgeting basics. Oh, and that last £20 – check your university's funding webpages for details of any crisis support.

> I get a bursary but have two children in nursery so spend a lot on childcare.

By now you'll be aware of the proposed changes to UK government funding of nursing and midwifery students. While before, your student bursary offered a 'pot of gold' to live on, the funding landscape for nursing and midwifery students may be subject to change, according to available budgets. So always check out updated information on your local authority website. Also, check out your university's funding webpages for any additional funding available to nursing and midwifery students, for example, from benefactors or dependants' allowances. Funds are limited and awards are competitive, so note the deadline and apply! You never know...!

Budgeting bullets:

- Open a student bank account – look out for the offers and incentives from banks.
- List your expenses, including the extras – placement, equipment, travel.
- Keep a spending diary.

- Increase your income – register for Agency healthcare work.
- Complete your HC1 form.
- Avoid library fines – set due date reminders.
- Buy second-hand textbooks.
- Save energy, lower your bills – switch off appliances.
- Smart shopping – look for the bargains, ask for a student discount, use vouchers.
- Get core software free through the university or discounted from suppliers.
- Clever cooking – freeze portions, e.g. day 1 meal plus day 2 lunch.
- Cheaper coffee/tea – buy a travel mug and make your own.
- Car share, cycle, walk, use public transport – remember student travel cards and pre-booked travel discounts.
- Childcare vouchers – check out providers and other budget-saving support.
- Night out – use your student card and vouchers; share a taxi home.
- Pay the 'need', save for the 'want'.
- Save the pennies, watch the pounds grow.

So note the help, bite the budgeting bullets and make it all add up! Oh go on, you know you want to!

DISABLED STUDENTS' ALLOWANCE – WHAT'S THAT?

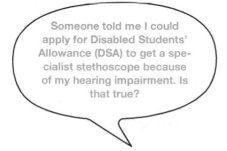

Someone told me I could apply for Disabled Students' Allowance (DSA) to get a specialist stethoscope because of my hearing impairment. Is that true?

Yes! DSA is additional government funding set aside for students who incur extra expenses over and above the average student because of their particular needs – a medical condition, disability or specific learning difficulty. See:

- www.nhsbsa.nhs.uk/
- www.saas.gov.uk/
- www.sfengland.slc.co.uk/
- www.studentfinancewales.co.uk/
- www.studentfinanceni.co.uk
- www.hea.ie/

It covers things like specialist equipment and software or one-to-one study skills support, with the support tailored to suit your specific need following a Needs Assessment discussion with a specialist Assessor. As with any public funds though, annual budgets and how they're allocated are subject to change, so always check your local funding authority regarding the application process and your eligibility. All applications are made through your Disability Service; so, if eligible:

- meet with your Disability Adviser
- submit the application
- have your Needs Assessment
- read and sign off your Needs Assessment report.

Once your application is approved and the DSA award letter received:

- arrange equipment delivery through the named company on your report
- follow up with software training
- arrange your study skills or other personal support through your Disability Service or named provider.

So money matters are dealt with, counted, managed! But when the full purse, empty wallet just doesn't add up, always check your university's online money guide. They're sure to have one! Learn how to manage your money at university and you'll learn how to manage it for life!

ACADEMIC SUPPORT

Reading a novel or writing a story isn't quite the same as getting to grips with academic work, so make the transition with your academic support service.

STRUGGLING WITH YOUR STUDIES?

Oh, don't you wish everything would run smoothly; you'd manage it all without any hiccups. But let's face it, at one time or another everybody who walks through the university doors needs academic support of some sort of another. It's a simple fact – we don't know it all; how could we? Sure we know how we like to study – or not study, and we think we know what works for us, but is it effective? Does it take account of our learning style (http:// vark-learn.com; Honey and Mumford 2001)? Is it balanced so we work efficiently between attending lectures, researching and writing up assignments, and our additional placement demands? More importantly, are we actually learning?

So what's your learning style? Note it, use it and make it work for you. Still a bit unclear about all this? Then revisit Activities 1.2 and 1.3 and check out your nursing and midwifery toolkit to see what works. Tried one, doesn't work so well? Then move on to the next one. Just mix and match different strategies until you've developed a personalised study skills toolkit that works for you. Understand your learning better? Then stick with it and create a mind map (https://bubbl.us; Arthur 2012) of how you like to work. Remember, learning should be enjoyable! Make it that way; make your learning style your learning strength and your motivation, and understanding should flourish.

> I've been away from education for 10 years and just found out I've got dyslexia. I'm a visual learner but am still struggling to keep up and manage assignments. I think I need some help.

Okay, a few things – get a study buddy; it helps to work with a fellow student in a situation where you feel comfortable mutually sharing experiences, ideas, smarter ways of working. Need a little more so you feel confident in what you're doing? Find one-to-one support works best? Then arrange individual study skills sessions tailored to your needs. There are two ways of doing this – through your academic skills advisers or your disability adviser, if you're eligible for DSA funding support.

With the age of technology and the academic and placement demands of nursing and midwifery programmes, universities are increasingly offering online study tutorials. You're expected to engage with your virtual learning environment to keep up to date with notes, discussions, tests, latest research, and what's on offer as support. So whether it's difficulties with resits, time management, referencing or drug calculations, check out the study skills workshops, drop-in sessions, online tutorials, online maths and drug calculation bitesize activities (www.bbc.co.uk/education), portable study apps and software, individual study sessions, and study buddy mentoring groups. Oh, and be open-minded when accepting feedback; it's a positive not a negative! Take the feedback, feed it forward and watch your skills improve.

Sorted out the practical study bits? Now what about the 'you' bits? Struggle with concentration, memory, anxiety, stress surrounding your studies? Then check out the workshops – stress management, mindfulness, confidence building, assertiveness training, or look at online support (Mental Health in Manchester, www.mhim.org.uk/helpguides/). Prefer to chat to someone confidentially, then arrange a counselling session. Your student counsellor will help you find the best way forward – from talking therapies to stress management to cognitive behavioural therapy, you'll find a range on offer in your university and your local area. Practical study bits and 'you' bits sorted – now for a few handy hints to make both bits work well.

LIBRARY

How often do we run around the library feeling stressed because we haven't a clue where to find exactly what we're looking for – that evidence-based article, the critical thinking book our tutor recommended, even the study skills book we need to help us understand referencing (Gribben 2012; Taylor 2012). And isn't all this searching worse when the deadline is slowly creeping up on us? It doesn't have to be this hard you know. So how can we actually enjoy our time in the library and put the fun back into researching information to learn new things? Two things really:

1. Always take time at the start of your course to get to know your library and your subject specific sections, including journals, books, reference works and online search engines.
2. Get to know your specialist librarian, learn the rules and regulations of the library, and take time to learn online searching procedures. It all pays off in the long run. Less stress, more success!

Oh, and if you've any specific needs ask about library support early on in your studies. So, for example, if you happen to be a slow reader because of your dyslexia or mental health condition, then it's time to liaise with your disability or counselling service and ask about loan extensions from the library or a library buddy. Support is available, you know. Ask too about accessing materials in alternative formats such as audio books or ebooks. Think – would any of this help support your learning? Yes! Then ask!

Taken the advice, spent some time learning the processes and the system? Let's see then how well you know your library and what it can offer.

ACTIVITY 2.3   REFERENCE SEARCH

Find the following – how long did it take you?

- Book on communication.
- Journal article on eating disorders.

(Continued)

(Continued)

- Online article on autoimmune neutropenia.
- Referencing guide used on your university's nursing and midwifery programmes.
- NMC standards on midwifery regulation.

How was that? Find these things easily enough? Mmm, could've been easier! Then join forces with your library buddy and create a personalised library system that makes using the library and learning in it fun! For example:

- allocate codes, e.g. A for article, B for book, JN for journal, etc.
- mind map and colour your subject sections
- colour your favourite library study corner.

Okay that's a few ideas for the library, but what about making technology work for us?

INFORMATION TECHNOLOGIST

Look let's face it, not all of us enjoy using technology or find it so easy, quite simply because we haven't grown up with it. It's all foreign to us and seems dauntingly complicated. If you struggle to find your way around computers then attend the technology workshops or get some one-to-one support so you can get to grips with the basics. Remember to back up your work regularly. We don't like the excuse that you've lost your work because you've forgotten to back it up, so make a habit of it. But if something goes horribly wrong and your laptop 'crashes' and you lose your work just as you're about to submit, then it's obvious – ask the experts for help. Don't waste time stressing when your technologist could be retrieving your work!

Waiting on some funding so you can buy a new laptop? Can't always manage to get into the computer lab? Then check out your university's loan system and borrow a laptop the way you'd borrow a book!

KEEP TRACK OF YOUR STUDIES

We all start out with good intentions, great plans to be that hard-working, curious student who manages it all – and then reality kicks in! Work piles up faster than we realise. But don't be too hard on yourself if things don't work the way you expect. It takes time to settle into student life, a new way of working, a new way of living. And with placements, work, study and assignments to juggle, things can quickly pile up. So take time at the start of your studies to plan your days and be diligent in managing your time, otherwise your time management at university may well become an unmanageable habit in practice. If that becomes the norm then you'll definitely need time to access some personal support.

PERSONAL SUPPORT

You're more than just a student; you've a life outside of university and placement – you know that. Things happen in life – you know that too, so when the going gets tough, access your SSFA for that much-needed personal and emotional support.

MANAGING STRESSFUL SITUATIONS

Let's face it – we all have stressful moments, situations, days, but how we deal with these makes the difference (www.nhs.uk/Livewell/studenthealth/Pages/Copingwithstress.aspx). Do we acknowledge it, do something positive about it and eventually manage it? Or do we keep running with it, hoping it all goes away, while eventually losing grip and tumbling further and further into a downward spiral?

ACTIVITY 2.4   LET'S ACT (ACKNOWLEDGE, CON-FRONT, TACKLE)

So you're stressed, let's acknowledge that – first step taken. But how do you confront it? Tackle it? Be honest! ACT – otherwise the stress goes on.

- Acknowledge what's stressing you.
- Confront its impact on your studies, placement and life.
- Tackle it to change the situation.

Ready to move forward? Let's identify key SSFA resources that can support you – counselling, funding, pastoral welfare, mentoring. What about other university or community resources? Ever considered mindfulness (Stone 2011) or yoga (Kollak 2009)? Shake off the stress, focus on success!

WHEN THE UNEXPECTED HAPPENS

It's all within your reach; shaping your academic success and ultimately your career. But, things can happen at any stage and what we see as the natural course ahead for us suddenly changes. The unexpected happens – family emergency, bereavement, sudden illness, financial struggles, placement difficulties – and the realisation that you're more than just a student hits home.

Up against that unplanned, unexpected situation? Spiralled into a crisis? Then support your physical and mental well-being by consulting your SSFA.

ACTIVITY 2.5   FIVE GOOD REASONS

Can you think of five good reasons for doing that? Pop them in a thought bubble!

They're yours; here are ours:

- Makes you feel better, less stressed and assured you're not alone; there's always someone who can help.
- Looks at the bigger picture and helps you put things into perspective.
- Guides you through the hard times; gets you over the hurdles and offers individual solutions to support your specific situation.
- Gives you the tools, confidence and courage to manage or change your situation.
- Lets you see that all things are possible; you can make it happen and achieve success.

Better to ask for help and advice at the start or early on rather than muddle your way through, stumble and fumble along and fall at the final hurdle, and not be in a position to register as a nurse or midwife.

MITIGATING CIRCUMSTANCES

So what are they, I hear you say? In a nutshell, these are unforeseen, unexpected or exceptional circumstances that have a negative impact on your studies and progression. So if you run into difficulty, contact your module leader or Personal Development Tutor/Director of Studies (PDT/DoS) and let them know your situation. It may well be you just need a week's extension to complete and submit your work. If it's more than this then check out and follow your university's mitigating circumstances process. Need advice and support with this? Then contact your Student Union or Student Services. They know the process and can point you in the right direction.

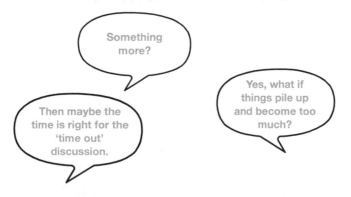

TAKING TIME OUT

It happens to the best of us. Things become too much and we need a break to avoid that potential breakdown. You know that one little thing sitting on our doorstep just waiting to come on in. So stop, suspend, survive! If it's a matter of completing your degree or not then do the sensible thing and take a break. Be assured, taking time out isn't so unusual today. In fact, it's more common than you realise. So don't stress about it all. If time out is just what you need, then take it – simple. Take some breathing space and come back refreshed.

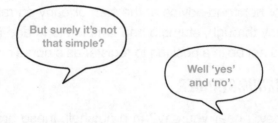

But surely it's not that simple?

Well 'yes' and 'no'.

Sure it can be hard making the decision to put things on hold for a while. You'll have many a sleepless night, tossing and turning, wrestling with the idea in your head, and feeling stressed, perhaps anguished about it all; not wanting to feel different, to feel as if you've failed – as if you're letting down yourself, others, those who believe in you. Deciding – honestly, that's the hard bit. But decision made, phew, a sigh of relief, a huge weight just lifted off your shoulders and so the rest seems simpler. Following the 'time out' process is the easy bit. That is, once you know how.

So how do I go about this? And what kinds of things do students take time out for?

Let's look at the issues a little more closely:

- what students take time out for
- making that decision
- the official process for interrupting your studies
- returning to your studies.

So to the first point – the single most common thing students takes time out for is stress. Yes, stress! Not because they necessarily suffer from anxiety as individuals or 'live on their nerves', but rather because of the worry of juggling more than one assignment alongside their practice learning placement, while dealing with family issues at the same time. Everything seems all too difficult – and 'coping' seems a foreign concept. Different people, different situations. So what's yours? Remember, before applying for time out, check with your university what's an acceptable mitigation (for example, sudden illness or pregnancy) and what's not (for example, planned holiday or stolen laptop before assignment deadline), and make sure your situation can be supported by another professional such as your GP.

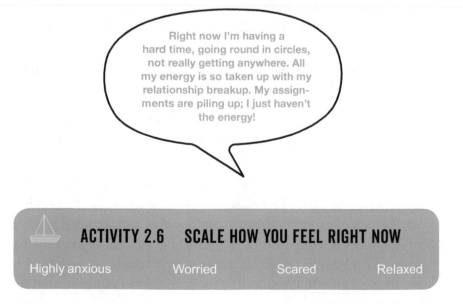

Right now I'm having a hard time, going round in circles, not really getting anywhere. All my energy is so taken up with my relationship breakup. My assignments are piling up; I just haven't the energy!

ACTIVITY 2.6   SCALE HOW YOU FEEL RIGHT NOW

Highly anxious   Worried   Scared   Relaxed

Can't see another way to get through the tough times other than taking time out? Talked it through with your family? Need some guidance from your SSFA? Then contact your Student Counsellor or Pastoral Support Adviser (www.nes.scot.nhs.uk/), if your university has one, and explore the personal issues related to your decision before dealing with any practical issues. It helps! Oh, and let them advocate on your behalf. Check out also the NUS' advice on practical issues such as funding (www.nus.org.uk/).

MAKING YOUR DECISION

You don't stand alone when making such an important decision, what's more you can't. Sometimes when you're in the thick of it, seeing the bigger picture is hard. You need others to help you do that and realise it's all possible – even after a break! So:

- Once you've discussed your situation and explored the question of suspending studies, chat with your PDT/DoS.
- Submit your application with all the relevant, supporting evidence.
- The School then considers your request, arrives at a decision, and notifies you in writing – generally within a few weeks.
- Your personal tutor advises you of what you can and can't do while on 'time out'.
- Returning? Then you'll need to know what to do next – again talk to your PDT/DoS.

'Time out' doesn't mean cutting yourself off from the university. While the idea is to be away from your studies and gather your strength again, some form of contact helps you realise it's only 'time out' not 'study time over'. So keep in touch with your PDT/DoS – whatever they're called – that academic staff member who follows your educational and professional development from day one of your studies. Regularly check in, tell them how you're doing, discuss your concerns and let them find a way forward for you so you'll return to your studies feeling prepared for what lies ahead.

RETURNING TO STUDIES

Unable to return at the agreed time? Have other unexpected things happened? Don't worry, just discuss further options with your PDT/DoS. Better to take extra time out than return too early, stress and fail. That's the 'unable' to return, now for the 'able to' return.

Feel the benefit of time out? Glad you made that decision? Ready to return? Then remember the checklist. Contact the following:

- your personal tutor to arrange a return to studies date
- your disability adviser to ensure your support is in place
- your school office.

A few practical things are worth noting – you generally can't ask for mitigating circumstances support retrospectively or undertake academic work during your time out. You might want to check whether 'time out' affects your access to the library and other university facilities. Oh, and also how your fees, bursary, loan and council tax exemption will be affected.

DISABILITY SERVICE

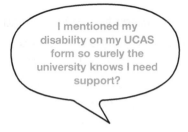

I mentioned my disability on my UCAS form so surely the university knows I need support?

Well, yes and no!

Don't assume your disability/dyslexia adviser automatically knows about your specific difficulty or your support needs. If you need exam allowances, adjusted on-campus accommodation, learning materials in alternative formats then register your needs with your

Disability Service – provide the evidence, discuss your needs and get your support. Oh, and sign the university's disclosure form protecting your data and giving permission to cascade your support needs to those who need to know, such as your exams team, lecturers, placement mentors. So what's on offer?

Support needs are individual and specific to you, and are generally four-fold (see Table 2.1).

Table 2.1　Support need examples

Support	Examples
Exams	Extra time, digital exam papers
General and/or inclusive support	Lecture notes in advance, networked assistive software
DSA	Assistive software, stethoscope, ergonomic aids
Placement	Protected time to administer medication for diabetes

Support decided, recorded, cascaded but still a few hiccups? Then chat to your School Disability Contact, i.e. the named person responsible for making sure you get all the support you need within the school. Not getting copies of notes in advance of the lecture so you can prepare and simply listen and engage with what's being taught? Then your school contact will ensure these are provided.

Still a hiccup? Got the specialist software and hardware through DSA? Want to use the university's networked software but not sure how it all works? Then make some time, arrange a training session with your assistive technology adviser and let technology work to your advantage (www.iansyst.co.uk, www.conceptnorthern.co.uk). If you're currently on placement, chat to your mentor and arrange an adjusted working schedule to accommodate this training. It's possible you know! So from getting your ideas down on paper with mind mapping, flashcard apps, storyboarding, to spellchecking, text to speech and speech to text processes, from recording to written assignment and referencing, through these sessions you'll learn smarter study strategies and minimise your student stress.

HEALTH AND WELL-BEING SERVICE

Worried about exams? Struggling with anxiety? Sleepless nights catching up with you? Stressing about assignments while managing placements and family commitments? Concerned you'll become another dropout statistic? And so, the stress bus has started on its journey, but where's your stop? Look, feeling some stress isn't a bad thing; how you manage it makes the difference. Not aware of your own stress? Then be aware!

While controlled stress (mindful in the moment – the *what is* situation) can boost motivation and performance in study, uncontrolled (in the imagination – the *what if* situation) can damage your health and well-being (Hassed and Chambers 2014). Let that continue and it can ultimately ruin your chances of completing your programme and achieving your goal, your dreams. So what's your preference? Okay, think! It's good to talk, is it not, to share concerns and experiences, and focus on the '*what is*' situation? Have you already organised a chat corner with your peers and shared similar stresses? Have you found that's not quite enough – other things are going on and you're still worrying and stressing? Then pause, breathe! Introduce mindfulness into your daily practices and tap into your SSFA a little more; make use of what's on offer; after all it's yours.

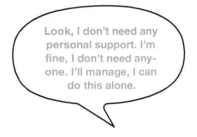

Look, I don't need any personal support. I'm fine, I don't need anyone. I'll manage, I can do this alone.

Look, you don't need to put on a brave face or even act tough. Nobody's expecting that. Just be yourself. Let's face it, how many nights have you tossed and turned, mulling things over in your head? Sleepless nights tossing and turning won't make the 'problem' disappear. Tackle it head on. Tapping into the support available should make the stress seem less intense; practising mindfulness should put a new perspective on things. Need help with a joint placement–university issue? Then talk to your Pastoral Support Adviser or PDT/DoS; they can advocate on your behalf. And if you feel overwhelmed, contact your Health and Well-being Adviser. Oh, and remember, make a note of all the out of hours services, such as Samaritans (www.samaritans.org/) or SANE (www.sane.org.uk/) – you never know when you just might need them.

COPING WITH THE EMOTIONAL BURDEN OF CARING

You're human; your patients are people – they're human too. And then there's their families – also human. You think and feel – emotions can be up, down, sometimes even raw. You deal with all theirs, you're professional, you've learned about communication, you've learned about boundaries and professional responsibilities and expectations, you can look at the bigger picture, somehow find the words to say the right thing, offer comfort and reassurance in difficult situations. That's the professional in you – but how do you channel your own emotions in the face of dealing with others' emotional and medical care so you don't reach 'burnout' (Shorter and Stayt 2010; Fearon and Nicol, 2011)? You're a midwife, you go on a journey with a mother from her first stages of pregnancy through to birth, all seems well and then things go wrong in labour. How do you cope?

Key to coping is giving yourself the space to reflect on your own needs within the situation (Johns 2013), and learning to talk about it with those with more experience. Allow others to help you create a meaningful sense of the situation. Your confidence will grow and your sense of compassion develop, so that coping with others' emotional experiences won't become your emotional burden.

PROFESSIONAL SUPPORT

Tapped into the university student support? Now for the professional support – skills, knowledge, practice – your professional questions answered in a nutshell.

SKILLS, KNOWLEDGE, PRACTICE – YOUR PROFESSIONAL QUESTIONS ANSWERED

It's a career, a profession, but careers advisers aren't the only people to give you professional advice.

Your placement mentor can be a valuable source of information; their personal experience, knowledge and expertise can be key in guiding you, even influential in helping you choose your career pathway. Stuck on a research project? Then ask your placement team for advice or some tips on smarter ways of working through assignments or with practical tasks on placement.

Not quite sure how to cope with the emotional burden of caring? Didn't expect your own emotions to surface in specific situations? Concerned about tackling a whistleblowing incident, even as a student? Then ask the professionals – your team, mentor, lecturer. Don't leave yourself exposed to unnecessary stress. Remember, early skill-forming and confidence-building makes for knowledgeable, compassionate, confident professionalism. Well, that's your placement mentor and your team but what's on offer in shaping your career?

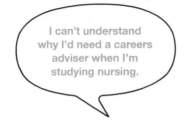

I can't understand why I'd need a careers adviser when I'm studying nursing.

Well why not? Listen, we all need careers guidance at some point in life. Even if it's just trying to sort out in our heads what's best for us in our working life. Sure you're going to be a nurse or a midwife, but what area of specialism? Neonatal, palliative, community, oncology, mental health – the list goes on forever! Think of the choice and the opportunities! You may still be a student but you're in the unique position where you can access advice to map out your career pathway step by step (Nursing Careers, http://nursing.nhscareers.nhs.uk/careers). So make the most of it! Don't wait until you're ready to graduate and register to practise. Ask for advice! Take the advice! Soak it all up! Well, why not?

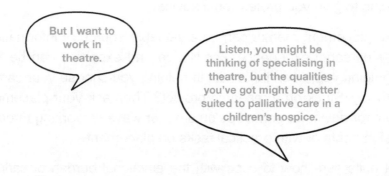

So explore your personal qualities, your strengths, communication and interpersonal skills and, importantly, your transferable skills, with your careers adviser.

Need to update your CV? Want to sell yourself well on paper and in interviews or presentations? Be assertive without seeming arrogant? Want to land that job or widen your employment opportunities? Then make use of what's on offer through your university careers service and check out Chapters 11 and 12 for more in-depth information and advice.

THOSE DREADED SURVEYS

Oh yes, there's always space in our lives for an appeal or complaint. We appeal if we're not happy with our mark, and we complain if things don't go our way. That's it, get it all out ... feel better then? It's all too easy to complain about the support and the services, and, of course, we'll quite happily do that in those end of year surveys. I'll soon tell them where they've gone wrong, I hear you say. Really?

Remember your feedback is important, so let's approach it constructively rather than destructively; your contribution to providing a more improved service is vital. So take a step back and ask – is there anything you feel they could have done differently? Something that would have made student life smoother and easier for you? Yes? Then tell them. But remember the positives too! How good would it be to let staff know you're grateful for their support.

TOP TIPS

✔ Identify your obligations and responsibilities.
✔ Organise your time to capture your day, week.
✔ Make a note of the support you need and store it alphabetically.
✔ Identify your advisers and the support they offer.
✔ Create a portable Student Support First Aider containing your key contacts.
✔ Complete your support processes using mind maps.
✔ Use a monthly budget planner.
✔ Attend study skills workshops.
✔ Work through study skills activities.
✔ Complete online study-related activities.
✔ Remember the 'me' time and participate in relaxation techniques/ workshops.
✔ Start shaping your career pathway and consider other options.
✔ Take time to get to know your library.
✔ Learn to use technology – attend the workshops.

So those are the tips, but don't forget your toolkit at the end of the book!

FURTHER READING

Breathing space: http://breathingspace.scot/
Cabellero, C., Creed, F., Goshmanski, C. and Lovegrove, J. (eds) (2012) *Nursing OSCEs: A Complete Guide to Exam Success*. Oxford: Oxford University Press.

Davey, L. and Houghton, D. (2013) *The Midwife's Pocket Formulary*, 3rd edition. London: Churchill Livingstone.

Frixione, N., Hettena, J. and Barnes, T. (2015) *Strategies for Coping with the Emotional Burden in Nursing*. Presentation: https://prezi.com/ltyveq5uvnnz/strategies-for-coping-with-the-emotional-burden-in-nursing/

Hutton, M. and Gardner, H. (2005) 'Calculation skills', *Paediatric Nursing*, 17(2). Middlesex: RCN Publishing Company.

Lapham, R. (2015) *Drug Calculations for Nurses: A Step by Step approach*, 4th edition. Boca Raton FL: CRC Press.

3 COMMUNICATION AND INTERPERSONAL SKILLS

⟹ Effective communication – the how, what, when and why
⟹ Verbal communication
⟹ Non-verbal communication
⟹ Written communication
⟹ Online communication
⟹ Communicating in difficult situations
⟹ Interpersonal skills – what they are
⟹ Positively communicating your values, beliefs and opinions
⟹ Problem-solving and decision-making

CHAPTER OVERVIEW

Communication is so much more than just what's said. It encompasses a whole range of activities, many subconscious, shared between two or more people – so-called interpersonal skills. To help you understand these skills, this chapter focuses on different styles of communication – verbal, non-verbal and written forms. It explores what effective communication looks, feels and sounds like, while considering potential barriers. It emphasises the responsibility of nurses and midwives to uphold professional standards of online communications, ensuring that any online activities maintain confidentiality and don't bring you or your profession into disrepute (NMC 2016). Finally, the chapter looks at the different relationships you'll form during your

(Continued)

(Continued)

training, showing you how to communicate in different ways with different people, in different situations. If you know how to do this, you'll confidently communicate your ideas while respecting others' contributions and values, even in difficult situations.

- Effective communication – the how, what, when and why
  - o Barriers to effective communication
- Verbal communication
- Non-verbal communication
- Written communication
- Online communication
- Communicating in difficult situations
- Interpersonal skills – what they are
  - o Your interpersonal relationships
- Positively communicating your values, beliefs and opinions
- Problem-solving and decision-making
- Top tips

EFFECTIVE COMMUNICATION – THE HOW, WHAT, WHEN AND WHY

You've been talking since you were two, right? You've made it through school, maybe even work, life in general, communicating fine so far, so why do you need to learn about communication now, I hear you say? Well, while you've been used to communicating in different environments before your student days, effective communication in the nursing and midwifery profession is fundamental to caring for people, and so it takes on a new importance in your life now. You need to know the how, what, when and why of this to ensure your communication is clear with no space for any misunderstandings.

Effective communication is that interaction between two people who share an equal part in the communication process, when the listener receives the message the sender intended to give. While the message itself is important, how it's sent and received is also part of effective communication, and so equally important. So how do we understand messages? Well, fundamentally we understand what people say in two ways:

- how they say things – the kind of terminology they use (easy or complex words), the speed, tone and pitch of voice.
- non-verbal gestures – eye contact, nods, smiles, frowns, touch and stance, whether arms or legs are crossed or an open posture is adopted.

Sounds a lot? Okay, let's see …

You want to be a nurse or a midwife – yes? And you want to understand why communication is so central to this profession – yes? Then I guess a good starting point is to check out the NMC standards for pre-registration midwifery education (2009) and nursing education (2010). This set of standards governs every undergraduate nursing and midwifery curriculum in the UK, providing guidance for the achievement of specific competencies and skills known as 'essential skills clusters' – core skills which must be achieved, including 'communication'.

By the end of your first year as a student, you're expected to communicate 'effectively so the meaning is always clear' (NMC 2009: 36; 2010: 110). This means clearly communicating with the patient you're caring for, whether they're a 5-year-old child, a 20-year-old woman or, indeed, a man in his 90s. You need to understand that the range of vocabulary, understanding and concerns of each of these patients will differ, and so you'll need to adapt your skills accordingly. But it doesn't stop there – you need to communicate with your patients' families, other professionals involved in their care, fellow nurses and midwives, your practice learning placement mentor, your lecturers and peers. And there's more. You'll be communicating in a variety of settings – university, people's homes, different hospital wards, outpatient clinics; with trauma, acutely ill or longer-term patients, with colleagues from social work, physiotherapists, and with primary care or third sector/ voluntary colleagues.

So how do you manage all this, and more importantly – how do you adapt? Well, with practise! There are many textbooks entirely dedicated to communicating and interpersonal skills – Peplau (1991), Bach and Grant (2011), and England and Morgan (2012), to name but a few. Of course, communication is such a fundamental skill that you probably don't really think about it except in situations when you realise it's all gone wrong. Those times when you realise you said something that negatively affected the other person or they said something that didn't feel quite right. Then you think, 'gosh, what went wrong'? We've all experienced this – but what do we do with our communication mishaps? Go on, tell me yours.

⛵ **ACTIVITY 3.1   COMMUNICATION MISHAPS**

Note one or two instances when your communication was clunky, when there was a misunderstanding or you reacted in a way you didn't intend to? How did the situation unfold? How did you 'make it right'?

Communication is a two-way process; we know that. In your personal interactions, both parties have a shared responsibility to 'get it right', whereas in your professional life, it's your responsibility. You need to ensure your message is clear, using language adapted to the situation. You need to listen to and hear what the other person is saying, observe their body language, interpreting it all in the moment – is what they're saying what they mean and how they feel? You also need to use non-verbal signs to show you're listening, such as making eye contact, smiling or simply nodding. And to ensure communication is effective, ask when things aren't quite clear for you, and, importantly, allow your patients (and others) to do the same. So be aware of what you'll look for so you'll know what information is correct and how to adapt your language and communication style, interpret body language and identify the difference between what the patient is saying and how they're actually feeling. How good is your communication awareness then? Let's check:

⚓ ACTIVITY 3.2 CASE SCENARIO

Consider the following. You're working with your mentor in a minor injuries unit when Nala brings in her 6-year-old daughter, Aisha, with a sore arm after falling from her bike. Aisha has been crying and Nala is worried, her voice is hesitant; she didn't see the accident. To assess Aisha's injury, you need to communicate effectively with Aisha and her mother. You need to find out information about the accident, how sore Aisha's arm is and then assess what treatment she needs. You start by introducing yourself; you smile. You ask Aisha questions she'll probably be familiar with answering – 'Are you six?', 'Can you wiggle your fingers?', 'Move your arm?' There's no visible wound. You encourage Aisha by saying 'well done', you nod, smile and then assure her that her arm is okay – 'Look it's working'. During the assessment, Nala becomes visibly less worried, she sits down rather than standing at the end of the bed, and rubs Aisha's leg. You document your assessment with support from your mentor, advising Nala and Aisha that the arm is probably sprained, and that paracetamol and rest should be all that's needed. You tell them it won't be long before Aisha is back riding her bike. When they leave they thank you.

Let's jot down the various interaction aspects in this scenario:

Introduction	
Communication skills	
Verbal information	
Non-verbal information	
Mother's body language	
Mother's voice	
How you adapted your language, and why	

Now let's look at the importance of these key features.

To make an assessment, you need to develop a trusting relationship between yourself and the patient, and in this case her mother. You do this by introducing yourself; as simple as this sounds, it's the first step in developing a therapeutic relationship and is extremely important. A campaign called 'Hello. My name is …', started in 2013 by Kate Granger, a doctor who was having treatment for cancer, emphasised the importance of this first step (http://hello-mynameis.org.uk). Kate's campaign has been so successful that healthcare staff now use this introduction; perhaps you've heard them. If you've not already used this phrase yourself, why not start adopting it now and see the difference it makes. 'Hello. My name is …' makes a good first impression!

You'll have noticed Aisha understood what she was asked to do, and could demonstrate the function of her arm by following your instructions and interactions. Take note though – there's a difference in how you'd ask a child and an adult to perform the arm movements; one example of adapting your language. By communicating verbally, supported by non-verbal nods, eye contact and positive noises, you can make a reliable assessment. You'll see that Nala is more relaxed when she comforts Aisha and rubs her leg. When Aisha and Nala leave, they reaffirm the communication was effective by thanking you. Finally, there's the written communication – a record of the assessment and the advice given.

Of course, you may not have noticed all these aspects of communication but hopefully we're giving you sufficient tools so you can start observing more, and evaluate your interactions when in practice. It's all part of the learning process and the job!

There are communication tools you can use as part of your practice, such as the SBAR tool – Situation, Background, Assessment and Recommendation (NHS Institute for Innovation and Improvement 2008). SBAR has been shown to reduce the incidence of miscommunication and is recommended for handover, between shifts and between professional teams. The tool offers a structure for handover so important information isn't lost. If you've not seen or heard of it before, check it out.

BARRIERS TO EFFECTIVE COMMUNICATION

While we've demonstrated effective communication in this scenario, many areas of healthcare are challenging for staff and students alike; such challenges can hamper communication. Let's see …

⛵ ACTIVITY 3.3   COMMUNICATION BARRIER

Consider the following scenario. It's the first time you've had to 'hand over' care at the end of a shift to another nurse or midwife. You're scared you'll forget something so you give the information as quickly as possible, trying not to use any tricky words that you might mispronounce. Your handover contains every detail of your patient's day, just to make sure nothing is omitted. You notice the person you're handing over to – who should be listening – is looking behind you, making you more nervous. You decide not to say anymore, so your mentor finishes the handover for you.

A few key points to help you understand what happened here:

- first time handing over care – inexperienced
- tried to give too much information, too quickly – anxiety levels rose
- no acknowledgement from receiver (nurse or midwife) during handover – they looked away
- no encouragement to continue with the handover – no engagement from the receiver; eye contact, nodding or smiling
- felt undermined and so stopped speaking.

How else could this scenario be interpreted? When the nurse or midwife looked behind you, they might have been looking at the patient to acknowledge them and assess whether your information 'fitted' with their appearance, and whether they looked well or poorly. It might not have been a negative reaction to your handover. Try to remember this as you communicate, as people's actions and behaviours can sometimes be misinterpreted (that's when we see the importance of non-verbal cues!). Don't worry – you'll learn this as you go along. And don't forget, mentors recognise that while handover is an important milestone in your education, it's difficult and also takes practice to master. So grasp the opportunity, tell your mentor if you're nervous, try to be self-aware, speak clearly and at a measured pace, identify and practise the key things you need to speak about, and confidently project the knowledge you've acquired from having cared for this patient during your shift, so the next member of staff can continue good patient care. Using the SBAR tool should help with the structure of the information you need to include for each patient's care you're handing over (NHS Institute for Innovation and Improvement 2008). Can you see how what's said, how it's said and the context in which it's said all affect the messages, which are given and received in different ways?

VERBAL COMMUNICATION

Okay, so what about other features of verbal communication? Let's face it, we've all been the subject of a standing joke! During my student days, I was in the clinical skills lab practising talking to a 'pretend' 5-year-old (you know, one of my peers sat in the bed). I said 'let's be rational about this' to the 'child'. Of course, that blunder became the standing joke for the remainder of my training. I mean, how many 5-year-olds in a hospital setting are going to be rational about anything? I was glad to have slipped up like that while practising my communication skills; trust me, I didn't make the same mistake again!

Yes, the words you choose play a big part in verbal communication but that's not all you need to think about. When giving and receiving information, the quality of information also depends on the amount you give. If, for example, you give too little information to your patient, you may find they're unable to make an informed decision; similarly, if you give too much, they may feel somewhat overwhelmed. If you're giving information to another healthcare professional and omit important details, this may affect your patient's care. The speed of information delivery is also important; speak too fast and you'll find some key words may be missed by your patient, their family or other healthcare professionals – this creates the potential for misunderstandings. So you see, there's so much more to verbal communication than you probably first realised.

NON-VERBAL COMMUNICATION

Non-verbal communication is just as important as what we say, as it accounts for more than half of all communication.

> **ACTIVITY 3.4 NON-VERBAL COMMUNICATION**
>
> Think about what these non-verbal actions tell us: crying, laughing, arms tightly crossed around your body, swaying, looking at the floor. Note it!

Looking at these on their own, it's difficult to know what these actions mean. Perhaps you've said crying is an emotional reaction to pain or grief, or it could also be relief, happiness, frustration or hopelessness. But how would you read this non-verbal cue while communicating? You could say the same about laughter, although it's not always associated with something funny. All of these non-verbal signs can be read in different ways. The context – what's going on – is important when trying to interpret other people's moods. Different cultures also come into play here.

The space people leave between each other while communicating, or the amount of eye contact they're willing to share varies from person to person, and culture to culture. While some people are comfortable with other people touching them, for example, others aren't. So be aware!

From your first days as a student, you'll need to understand how your non-verbal communication impacts upon the person you're talking to, and similarly how to interpret their body language. So observe and learn! Do this and before long you'll confidently be able to acknowledge that you've noticed their behaviour, and even feel that you can open up an avenue for them to discuss their feelings:

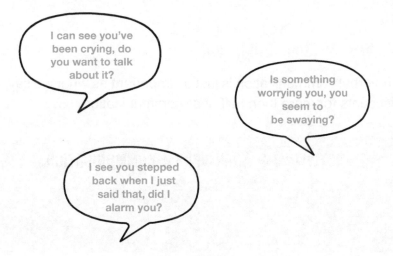

Of course, all this takes practice too. Learn and understand the non-verbal role of communication and you'll soon learn to combine verbal and non-verbal forms of communication, allowing you to actually get to know the other person, rather than making assumptions about how you think they're feeling.

WRITTEN COMMUNICATION

So have you already written your first assignment or documented care in a patient's notes? Not yet? Don't worry, you'll soon get used to the two different styles of communication. In written assignments, such as essays, the thoughts you convey will be supported by references to others' ideas and opinions – more on this in Chapter 6. In clinical practice though, written communication is different. Many trusts use handwritten notes, although some use electronic patient records. The principles of both are that the notes are contemporaneous (written as soon as possible after the event). When you write up a patient's notes, you only need to describe exactly what's happened during your shift, you need to be objective and factual and write clearly, using black pen.

So how do you learn to write case notes using all this strange medical language? Well, on the job really! There are some commonly agreed abbreviations in nursing and midwifery practice, which you'll learn as you progress through the different placements. However, the main thing to remember is that all written communication about patients and any related activity form a legal document, which can be referred to, if necessary, in a court of law. That's why it's so important to think carefully about what you write and how you write it – refer to the NMC record-keeping guidance within The Code (NMC 2015a); always state the facts without interpretation, and make sure your signature is printed and clear.

In addition to being a legal requirement, the nursing or midwifery records are also a way of letting other professionals know what's happened while caring for your patient. If you forget to document any of this then it looks as though some care has been omitted, or not given.

Don't worry, your placement mentor will support you while writing up your notes, helping you to develop your reporting skills. They'll also counter-sign your notes to show they've read and agree with your entry (or the care given).

ONLINE COMMUNICATION

No doubt, you'll communicate with others online during the course of your studies – sending emails to your tutors or peers, posting on your cohort's closed Facebook account, actively engaging in Twitter or even making YouTube clips. These are great ways to communicate and keep learning interesting by sharing ideas with other like-minded people, and for discussing professional concepts such as compassion, while generally broadening your horizons, don't you think? Be mindful though of the NMC *Social Media Guidance* (2016). Be aware also that the debate surrounding social media, and whether it's good or bad for the nursing and midwifery professions, takes many avenues (Jones and Hayter 2013).

Questions have been raised about whether students, especially those beginning their training, fully understand what's an appropriate post or tweet and what's not. Younger students in particular, who've grown up using social media, may not fully appreciate that privacy settings aren't 100 per cent private, and that a silly mistake can cost their career. So while you acknowledge the positives of online communication, be aware of the negatives – the consequences if you unwittingly:

- breach patient confidentiality
- share information about others without their consent
- post inappropriate comments about patients, colleagues or the Trust you work in
- do anything that breaks the law.

Remember, you've a duty to protect the public, your professional self and your profession, even as a student, so familiarise yourself with the NMC guidelines for using social media (see Chapter 9). All good steps in the learning process!

ACTIVITY 3.5   SOCIAL MEDIA COMPLEXITIES

Let's consider the two complexities of social media. What would you do if a patient tries to contact you via Facebook, or if photos of you singing in a rowdy bar suggesting you're drunk are posted online? Want some food for thought? Then note them in a thought bubble.

Some advice:

- Patient contact online – this should be declined even though you may feel a little awkward when you next meet them. However, explaining that professional boundaries are clearly stated by the NMC should help the situation.
- The photo scenario – it's most likely a friend who posted your image. Simply ask them to remove it (but remember things are never totally removed from social media once posted!), explain your professional guidelines on social media and the potential consequences of breaching them, and ask them not to post anything potentially compromising again.

COMMUNICATING IN DIFFICULT SITUATIONS

I'm sure, even as a student, you've some patients under your care experiencing difficult situations – bad news they need to consider, an unexpected or life-changing diagnosis, a pregnant woman or new mother who's been told her baby has an abnormality or won't survive. Being fairly new to the profession, you'll undoubtedly find this hard to deal with personally, but bear in mind your role is also to support the person you're caring for. And while it won't be your place to give the news, you'll need to listen to the patient mull this news over or talk about their feelings and thoughts.

Sometimes when people are in difficult situations they become stressed and may communicate in a loud and aggressive way. Your role here isn't to exacerbate the situation but rather to diffuse it. If you're new to dealing with these kinds of situations, it's best to observe and ask your mentor for advice and support. In fact, The Code (NMC 2015a) insists you do this: 'ask for help from a suitably qualified and experienced healthcare professional to carry out any action or procedure that is beyond the limits of your competence'. Once you're more experienced, you'll be able to deal with such situations in a supportive manner by explaining, reassuring or acknowledging the issues which are causing your patient concern.

Whatever the situation, it's important to be honest and factual and not raise hopes or expectations about actions to resolve matters when you can't be sure of the outcome. Take the example of dealing with an emergency situation – you may need to explain to patients and their partners or family members what happened. Initially, of course, your mentor will do this, but as you become more senior you may take on this role. Even if your mentor does explain the situation, the person you're caring for may want to ask you about their emergency to make sense of it. You can help by listening and reinforcing what your mentor said, or getting advice if the person hasn't understood at all. Asking for help/advice is another part of your learning process.

Another common difficult situation is communicating with people who may not speak English. You may well know you should have an interpreter and not use family members to translate care options and choices, but in this situation right now, you've no other choice. Sure, you can get by on some sign language and maybe even a translation app on your phone, but you may have to rely on others to translate for you as well. This isn't ideal, not for you nor the person you're caring for. It may lead to misunderstandings or care choices not being offered well, so try to arrange an appropriate interpreter or use Language Line as soon as you can, to ensure your patient receives the same level of care and communication as others.

INTERPERSONAL SKILLS – WHAT THEY ARE

Okay, we've considered how information is communicated, but what about how interpersonal skills are used in that communication – your interaction with others? What are these interpersonal skills exactly? Well, they're skills such as verbal and non-verbal communication, listening, negotiating, problem-solving, assertiveness and decision-making; all key in nursing and midwifery communication. Think of your interpersonal skills as your 'professional friend'; they're transferable to nursing and midwifery. Develop your skills and learn to support them to work through issues, just as you would a personal friend. With friends, we tend to choose people whose personalities we like and so we often find it easier to communicate with them. Yet, in your professional role, you'll have to communicate effectively with people you may not be keen on, whether these are members of staff, relatives, or occasionally, dare I say it, a patient.

In your professional role, you'll still need to demonstrate empathy, compassion and respect for others' choices and decisions, regardless of whether you agree or like them. Perhaps it's in these circumstances that interpersonal skills come most to the fore. One old but relevant theory of nursing that applies equally to midwifery is Peplau's (1991) four-step interpersonal relations theory, which considers nursing as a therapeutic interpersonal process between the patient and nurse, with the common goal of promoting well-being:

1. Orientation – when the two sides engage, the nurse or midwife provides explanations, information and answers questions.
2. Identification – as the relationship develops, the patient expresses feelings to the nurse or midwife, and the two work more closely together.
3. Exploitation – when the patient trusts the nurse or midwife and makes full use of the services offered.
4. Resolution – when their relationship ends.

So let's consider these four steps in relation to those you'll have relationships with during the course of your training.

YOUR INTERPERSONAL RELATIONSHIPS

The first people you're likely to meet are your peers; fellow students on your programme. While some will become lifelong friends, there will be others whose opinions you may not agree with and some you probably won't get on with. Regardless of any differences, you've a responsibility, as a nursing and midwifery student, to always communicate respectfully in all contexts – university, in practice learning placement and online. After all, this is what's expected of a true professional! No less!

Other people you'll develop relationships with are your PDT/DoS and practice mentor. Both are there to support, guide, teach and assess you. The nature of these relationships is very different, even though their roles are similar. While you'll see your PDT/DoS individually, you may also go to them with a problem or for a termly review. Your mentor, on the other hand, will usually only have you (and possibly another student) to work with, so you'll possibly build a closer relationship with these people. Depending on the area of practice you're in, you'll either be working in close contact on a one-to-one basis with your mentor, for example, in the community setting, or in a team situation on a busy ward, in an outpatient department, in a booking-in clinic or in a rehabilitation setting. The strength of your relationship will change depending on the context, as you follow Peplau's (1991) theory – build (orientate), affirm (identify), utilise (exploit) and end (resolve) your interpersonal relationships with your mentors in different areas, in different ways throughout your training. The purpose of exposing you to these different relationships is to enable you to become more independent as you approach the end of your training, and become a qualified nurse or midwife.

The interpersonal relationships with your patients are also dependent upon a number of additional factors – the length of time you spend with them, the amount of care they need and how much you personally provide, and when and where they go after their care episode is over. While you may develop deep, personal connections to your patients, you need to be aware at all times that you're their nurse or midwife – a professional, and not their friend. By this we mean you've a responsibility to maintain professional boundaries, which can be difficult, especially when you're building therapeutic and enabling relationships with the people you're caring for. The Code (NMC 2015a: 15) is very clear on this – 'stay objective and have clear professional boundaries at all times with people in your care (including those who have been in your care in the past), their families and carers'.

POSITIVELY COMMUNICATING YOUR VALUES, BELIEFS AND OPINIONS

In university, you'll have the opportunity to discuss your values, beliefs and opinions verbally and in writing in your assignments. Some people will agree with your thoughts, others may not. Depending on how much experience you already have of people challenging your beliefs, this can feel awkward. However, much can be learned from acknowledging and discussing differences. Remembering to listen to the other person's perspective is really important – in fact it's one of the fundamental aspects of effective communication, as is not interrupting them. You don't have to agree with everyone and you're allowed different points of view, but so are they.

In practice, you may have different opinions from others in your team. You still need to work with these team members, so keep all communication between you respectful and find a way to resolve your differences, away from the patient area. While you're at work you may need to be more flexible in your views and come to a compromise, especially if you remember that you're both there to improve patient care, health and well-being. In some cases, you may need to agree to disagree, but you still have to provide good quality care together. With patients, you should respect their wishes even if they don't align with your own values.

PROBLEM-SOLVING AND DECISION-MAKING

All the above communication styles and techniques when combined can help you make decisions and solve problems. Look back at Activity 3.2, on Aisha's care. You can see that you used communication skills to assess how badly Aisha was injured. By asking open-ended questions such as 'Tell me about what happened' and listening to the response while watching a person's body language, you can assess the extent of the problem. Initially,

Aisha's body language might have been closed, as she crossed her good arm around her sore one. As she relaxes and responds to your encouragement and instructions she may become less frightened of the injury and her posture becomes more open. In this way, you can problem-solve through her injury and make decisions about the care she needs.

Whatever care you're undertaking in clinical practice, you use communication skills to assess, plan, discuss and implement the necessary actions to help your patient. These include a range of verbal, non-verbal and written communication strategies. You'll learn more about these on your programme in theory, and practise the skills and interpret their meanings in practice. You're not expected to know everything all at once; your programme is three or four years long after all. You'll incrementally build up your communication range and strategies as a student, and you'll continue to develop these once you're qualified. So get communicating!

TOP TIPS

✔ Stand back at a social event and watch people's body language. Are some people leaning in towards others, or standing more awkwardly, perhaps with their arms crossed? Think about what this tells you and look out for this body language in your professional practice.

✔ If allowed, bring home blank documentation from work so you can practise writing on it.

✔ Read the NMC Social Media Guidance, especially if you use it.

✔ Think about whether you could separate your personal and professional accounts, discuss this with your peers.

So, those are the tips, but don't forget your toolkit at the end of the book!

FURTHER READING

'Art of good communication': http://journals.rcni.com/page/ns/students/clinical-placements/patientcentred-care/art-of-good-communication

Byrom, S. and Downe, S. (eds) (2015) *The Roar Behind the Silence: Why Kindness, Compassion and Respect Matter in Maternity Care*. London: Pinter & Martin Ltd.

Pavord, E. and Donnelly, E. (2015) *Communication and Interpersonal Skills*, 2nd edition. Banbury: Lantern Publishing.

Sully, P. and Dallas, J. (2010) *Essential Communication Skills for Nursing and Midwifery*, 2nd edition. Edinburgh: Mosby.

4 PROCRASTINATION: PUTTING THINGS OFF AND DELAYING THE OBVIOUS

⟹ Procrastination – what is it exactly?
⟹ The five-step Getting into Gear process

🔭 CHAPTER OVERVIEW

This chapter deals with that little thing we're all good at – putting things off until tomorrow. In our daily dealings with our studies and placements, we fumble around grappling to get things done and move forward but somehow we can't; we keep putting things off. In a nutshell – we procrastinate! By taking you through the five-step Getting into Gear process, this chapter will help you face your procrastination habits, find ways to break the mould, and develop strategies that work for you so that - tomorrow does come, and the job gets done.

- Procrastination – what is it exactly?
- The five-step Getting into Gear process

  o Step 1: Identifying yourself – what type of procrastinator are you?
  o Step 2: Naming your procrastination pattern
  o Step 3: Taking ownership
  o Step 4: Making the change
  o Step 5: Reviewing the change

- Top tips

PROCRASTINATION – WHAT IS IT EXACTLY?

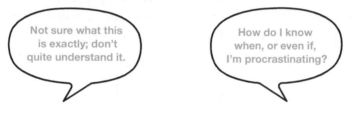

Not sure what this is exactly; don't quite understand it.

How do I know when, or even if, I'm procrastinating?

Okay let's put it this way – you've an essay to write and it's hard getting your ideas down on paper because you've so many notes: what do you do? When you're trying to manage a number of issues on placement, plus personal commitments and assignments to submit, what do you do? Get yourself organised and get started, or 'run away', thinking that you'll get it sorted out at some point or another, so there's nothing much to worry about. But at which point? Oh, I'll do it tomorrow, I hear you say. And so one day runs into the next and then the next, and that 'tomorrow never comes' habit creeps in and takes hold. So, in a nutshell, we should but we don't, and we've a new friend – procrastination (Kelly 2007). And oh, how we love this friend. It's been part of us for so long, we're comfortable with it and we certainly don't want to get rid of it. However, we really must!

So let's be realistic then – in trying to manage practice learning placements, assignments, and even sometimes a family, you simply can't afford to have a 'tomorrow never comes' moment! And in student life something always suffers – generally your assignments. Leaving things to the last minute, you run out of time, stress sets in and you adopt that 'just get anything down, oh, that'll do' attitude; your deadline at least is met (Tefula 2014) – relax, phew! But what's the outcome?

I admit, breaking the habit is hard; it's part of who we are and so getting rid of that 'friend' isn't easy. But to manage both your studies and your placements effectively and to make them stress-free don't just seize the day, be mindful in seizing the moment (Hassed and Chambers 2014), and honestly reflect on your current procrastination practice; what you do and why.

Well, does it all work for you or are you always trying to catch up? Note it! Have you discovered anything you could do differently? Note it! Have you managed to gather a few ideas then? Or are you even procrastinating about that?

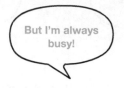

Sure you are; nobody disagrees with that. Procrastinators are always busy but with the wrong things (Tefula 2014). If I'd a penny for every time I cleaned my oven instead of polishing off my assignment, I'd be a millionaire? How true is that for you?

Okay, let's get serious here and do a little procrastination health check; that should make things clearer. Now we'll embark on the five-step Getting into Gear process, ready to admit our habits and start changing our behaviours (Gribben 2012).

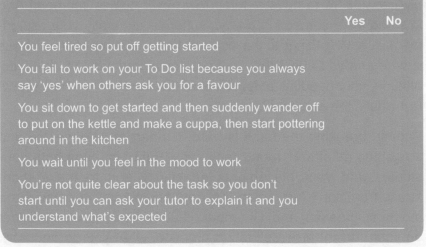

⚓ ACTIVITY 4.1 PROCRASTINATION HEALTH CHECK

How healthy is your procrastination? Add a tick to the Yes or No column for each statement.

Table 4.1 Procrastination health check

	Yes	No
You feel tired so put off getting started		
You fail to work on your To Do list because you always say 'yes' when others ask you for a favour		
You sit down to get started and then suddenly wander off to put on the kettle and make a cuppa, then start pottering around in the kitchen		
You wait until you feel in the mood to work		
You're not quite clear about the task so you don't start until you can ask your tutor to explain it and you understand what's expected		

	Yes	No
You find it hard getting your ideas down on paper so need some mind-map training to help you manage		
You keep waiting for the perfect time to get started		
You talk your way out of starting as your life is so busy with more fun things you enjoy		
You wait until the deadline is looming and then think about getting started		
You don't particularly enjoy the subject, aren't particularly motivated and so struggle to get started		
You're afraid of failing and being judged and so you keep delaying getting started		
You feel overwhelmed trying to juggle placement, assignments and personal life, and feel stuck		
You start strong and feel in control, but then lose your way because you're disorganised		
You're not quite sure what's expected in the learning outcomes and you keep putting off asking for advice to make them clearer		
You underestimate the time needed to complete the assignment and haven't planned your time effectively		
You underestimate how difficult the task is and you don't ask for help		
You have a 'let's wait for tomorrow' attitude		
You whine, grumble and complain about writing assignments rather than tackling them one at a time		
You feel guilty about procrastinating but don't do anything about it		
You can't get past the introduction because you want it all to be perfect and so keep re-writing it		

What's your health check telling you? If you've answered 'yes' to more than half of these then it's time for change, don't you think? So for you, which one is it? Follow the process – taste success? Ignore the process – experience endless stress?

THE FIVE-STEP GETTING INTO GEAR PROCESS

Procrastination isn't something that's suddenly just happened to you; it's been lurking there all the time; part of your very DNA and you're so well practised you haven't even noticed it! And what's more, there's no magic button to suddenly make it disappear.

Don't get me wrong, it's not going to be easy, particularly when juggling many different things at the same time; pressure soon builds up and stress levels rise. But at some point you need to test your belief about your commitment to your nursing or midwifery studies, face your fears, move out of your comfort zone, and get back on track so you enjoy your learning rather than constantly stressing about it. Want to 'walk the walk' as well as 'talk the talk'? Then follow the five steps set out here and you'll surely get there. Oh, and be honest; otherwise there's no point.

STEP 1: IDENTIFYING YOURSELF – WHAT TYPE OF PROCRASTINATOR ARE YOU?

So let's be clear about what you'd like to achieve. You've come into nursing or midwifery as a career option. What's your end goal and how do you intend to get there? You start of full of enthusiasm; classes are interesting and you can't wait until your first placement. You feel you're learning a lot, you're organised, motivated, keeping on top of it all, and you're happy you've made a great start. Correct? And you plan to continue working like that so everything will be plain sailing. Correct? So, let's define your goals – look backwards to move forwards.

> ⚠️ **ACTIVITY 4.2   GOAL PLAN?**
>
> You want to be a nurse or a midwife – why this profession? Frame it … summarise your goal in the circle below.

Ask yourself – what kind of student do you want to be? What kind of practitioner? Now, using Table 4.2 as a guide, tell me how you plan to achieve this?

Table 4.2 Goal plan

End goal (what you want to achieve)	Qualify as a knowledgeable, skilled and professional practitioner
Mid-point (how you plan to get there)	Where do you like to study best (e.g. library)? How do you like to study (e.g. background music)? Who will help you (e.g. study buddy)?
Start off (how you step out into university)	Motivated, well organised, excited, you start your studies full of beans!

Feel good seeing your responses? Let this define your learning and your practice; remember this during the hard times. Goals defined, health check done – now gauge your procrastination temperature.

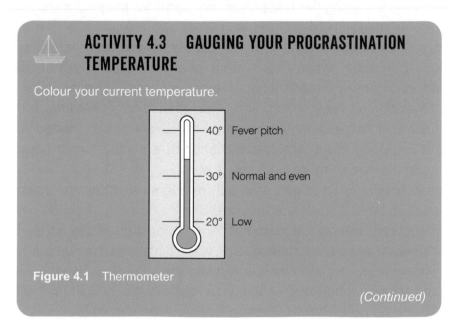

⚓ ACTIVITY 4.3   GAUGING YOUR PROCRASTINATION TEMPERATURE

Colour your current temperature.

—40° Fever pitch

—30° Normal and even

—20° Low

Figure 4.1 Thermometer

(Continued)

(Continued)

fever pitch = stressed, constantly worried, guilty and not very confident

normal and even = fairly organised and on top of things, reasonably motivated

low = relaxed, confident, focused, motivated and hard-working

Okay, step back now and reflect. Which temperature is most positive and favourable for you?

CASE STUDY

Dithering Daisy (yes, that's what she's called!) has recently moved into university accommodation but kept on her part-time job from home. Daisy has just started her first surgical placement. She's excited about moving from the classroom to the ward; maybe getting a chance to see how things work in the operating theatre. Even though she's always better with practical things than academic assignments, she wasn't too worried about completing her first placement portfolio; keeping a record of everything she'd learned and what she felt she still had to learn. She was keen to do well on placement, but there was one part Daisy wasn't quite clear about and she kept putting off asking her mentor's advice, thinking it would sort itself out. Re-writing an assignment didn't worry her too much either; her tutor told her exactly where she'd failed and what needed to be improved, so it was just a matter of a simple tweak here, a simple tweak there and she'd surely pass. She still had a few months or so to sort it all out, re-submit and get that pass; enough time – or so she thought. She came home from placement tired, stressed, deflated; it hadn't been a great day and her confidence had been dented. She wasn't interested in doing any written work, but one day had run into the next, and then weeks and months, and the deadline was looming, but still she put off getting started. That's Dithering Daisy – I wonder why!

What type of procrastinator is Daisy? And you? Find that out and you'll have taken that first small step towards breaking the mould. Why not take another step forward and jot down a few strategies to break through this; we've given you a few ideas in Figure 4.2.

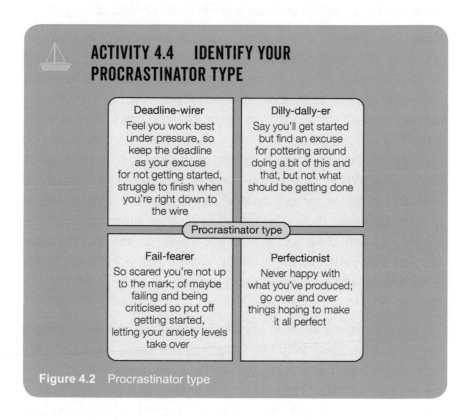

ACTIVITY 4.4   IDENTIFY YOUR PROCRASTINATOR TYPE

Deadline-wirer
Feel you work best under pressure, so keep the deadline as your excuse for not getting started, struggle to finish when you're right down to the wire

Dilly-dally-er
Say you'll get started but find an excuse for pottering around doing a bit of this and that, but not what should be getting done

Procrastinator type

Fail-fearer
So scared you're not up to the mark; of maybe failing and being criticised so put off getting started, letting your anxiety levels take over

Perfectionist
Never happy with what you've produced; go over and over things hoping to make it all perfect

Figure 4.2   Procrastinator type

If you identify with one of these then you're definitely a procrastinator – so which one are you? Can you think of a strategy to break through this? How about capturing your ideas? Saying 'No' to helping others with irrelevant tasks? Starting small, planning what can be done quickly? If you're not any of these but maybe a different type of procrastinator, check out Appendix 4. If you're more than one of these and your temperature is currently around fever pitch then it's time for real change! So let's accept some responsibility for your learning and your procrastinating ways. Nobody can do this for you, so tackle the things that are blocking you head-on. Do it now, not tomorrow! Not sure how? Need some help to get started? Let's take a step back and reflect on Daisy's story again. Is it clear why her friends call her 'Dithering Daisy'? What could she have done differently to make the end result more positive, reduce her stress levels and increase her confidence? Is there anything positive you can learn from this? Note it!

Now think back to a time when you found yourself in a similar situation. Who supported you then and what small things worked for you? Did they make a difference to creating a more achievable, less overwhelming situation, making you feel more confident in moving forward with a more manageable and productive working pattern? Lots of questions I know – but overall, did you do well on placement? Did you achieve a great grade rather than the accept-able one you'd become so used to – just scraping by because of that lifelong friend 'procrastinator' (Ackerman and Gross 2005)? More importantly, did this great grade change how you approach your work? Yes, but it was short lived, I hear you say. What's that – you fell into your old ways again? Don't worry! Hold on to the good feeling and positive working pattern it gave you, and simply start again. No harm in that – just get back on track!

Working out strategies that work for you and your learning style is key to your success (http://vark-learn.com). Make a note of what positively supported you in your earlier experience, and eliminate the things that didn't help. Then mix and match the aids in your nursing and midwifery toolkit, pull the resources together and plan small steps; those daily, short, sharp, 10-minute tasks that you feel are achievable, manageable and actually enjoyable. It may be small but this is the first step in helping you find a support strategy that should ultimately enable you to finally break the mould. I know it's only the first step but it's an important one.

STEP 2: NAMING YOUR PROCRASTINATION PATTERN

Identified and named it? Now let's frame it and shame it. It's not easy I know, but naming is the first step to reframing it. So let's look honestly at the things that hold you back from getting started. Remember, you're not alone on this professional journey; make the process easier by working with others on the Buddy Billboard activity. A word of caution though, don't form a group full of like-minded procrastinators; that would be counter-productive – you'd only end up procrastinating about your procrastination habits, and you'd be continuously stuck. So, gather a mix of people to make things work – listen to how others approach their work, reflect on your own approach and generate new discussion so you can learn to manage your procrastination moments better.

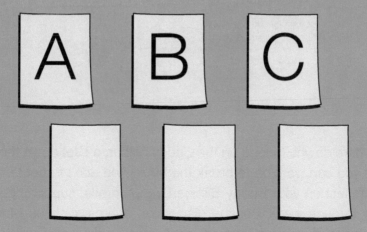

ACTIVITY 4.5   BUDDY BILLBOARDING

In your study group, create a floor-size Buddy Billboard. Of course, we couldn't leave him bare so we've created some ABC cards (Fig.4.3) as an example to help you name your procrastination habit and see where you fit on Buddy BillBoard.

Figure 4.3   ABC cards

A-cards: Approach, apply yourself, avoidance, awareness, attack, achievable, assess, accomplishment, accountability, affected, afraid, admit, attitude

B-cards: Belief in self, bits and pieces, beat it, bounce back, blocks, breakdown barriers, buddy work, better, believable reasons, bite the bullet, balance, besides

(Continued)

(Continued)

C-cards: Control, confidence, change, cure, cope, calmer, convince yourself, commitment, consequence, chunk it, can do

So place the cards face down in the middle of the table and choose one. Then share something about the word you chose in relation to your procrastination habits, e.g. 'approach' – explain your approach to assignments. It could be something positive or negative.

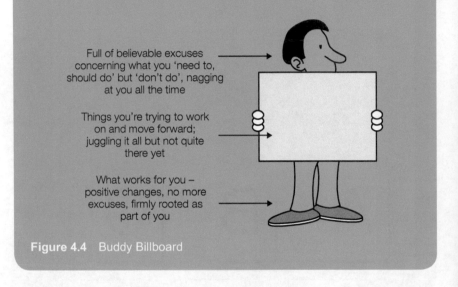

Full of believable excuses concerning what you 'need to, should do' but 'don't do', nagging at you all the time

Things you're trying to work on and move forward; juggling it all but not quite there yet

What works for you – positive changes, no more excuses, firmly rooted as part of you

Figure 4.4   Buddy Billboard

So where do you belong on the Buddy Billboard? Jot down the one thing you can work on to break the habit. And don't forget to regularly reflect on your Buddy Billboarding progress, supporting each other through weekly online discussion boards such as Moodle; remember, if using a non-university secure discussion room be mindful of the NMC *Social Media Guidance* (2016). Work hard to maintain this support so that you continue your professional journey together and achieve your goals.

Still need a helping hand? Then why not start moving forward, taking ownership of your procrastination by jotting and plotting what you need to do now on Buddy Billboard, and add some motivating slogan cards too, for example:

- Change is possible.
- Stay motivated, reach your goal.
- Get organised, stay organised.
- A little at a time means progress.
- Stop procrastinating today, not tomorrow.
- There's no time like – well, how about now!

Procrastination – having established *how* we do it, let's break the mould. Whether it's software from your toolkit or a hard copy paper version, create your own 'weekly duties' timetable – lectures, seminars, tutorials, placements, school run, family commitments, library time, social time – and stick with the calendar. Write your To Do list and prioritise tasks.

Answer honestly, admit your procrastination type and shake off the pretence; otherwise you're only kidding yourself. If you can't, then you need to ask – why am I really here studying nursing or midwifery? Keep the goal in mind!

STEP 3: TAKING OWNERSHIP

The reasons we find for procrastinating are as much a part of us as the very art of procrastination itself. We never fail to surprise even ourselves with yet another new-found excuse, or reason as we like to call it. A reason sounds nicer, don't you agree? But really procrastination is pure, plain and simple – putting off the inevitable and delaying the obvious (Tefula 2014).

Taking ownership means you've:

- admitted to habitually putting off things
- identified and named your procrastination habit
- acquired a general sense of your student-practitioner life as a procrastinator
- accepted that you want to do something positive to break the habit
- taken the first step to change.

So what's your believable reason for avoiding all this?

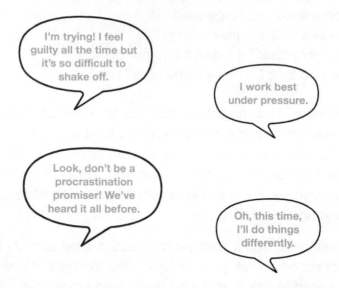

Sure you will – but do you ever really? Stop kidding yourself and knuckle down! Take ownership and get into gear now with that first small step; not tomorrow – now! And while you're doing that recognise what's going on in your life elsewhere; what's not working and needs to be tackled. Shake off the guilt, break through your perfectionist attitude; these things only drag you down, waste more time and encourage more procrastination (Hassed and Chambers 2014). Get support and talk about it all; it's all there in your SSFA (Chapter 2). Face your fears!

ACTIVITY 4.6   MIRRORING JANUS

Think of two situations in your everyday life: one where you've put things off, another where you've tackled things head on. Mirroring Janus will let you see that you're both part of the problem and part of the solution. Just as the problem lies within you, so does the solution (Gribben 2012). Be open and honest in your response.

Table 4.3 Mirroring Janus	
What I put off	
What I tell myself	
Consequences	
How I feel about this	
What I could change and how	
	What I tackle
	What I tell myself
	Benefits
	How I feel about this
	What I could improve upon

Note the difference in your mirror responses – your personal situation, attitude, goals, support, reward? Do you experience more confidence, less stress? What about your student life in university and placement? These are your problems and so your solutions; doodle what you've learned and can do differently. Which do you prefer – the put off or the tackled? Which one makes you feel less anxious and more in control? What are the consequences of not doing the work or the benefits of doing it? Reflect on that when you delay things!

Now – your To Do list. Are you prioritising? Aiming for a positive, upward spiral where you're empowering yourself and your self-esteem is boosted? Are you doing one thing daily to get that guilty procrastination feeling to become a thing of the past? Yes, no? Get started! Can't you see that the longer you take to get started on something, the harder it is to work on or even complete? It eats into your other time, panic sets in and you do that guilty 'all-nighter' right before the deadline; results are poorer than you'd like or are capable of achieving (Hassed and Chambers 2014). Are you actually being fair to yourself or your profession?

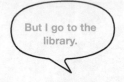

But I go to the library.

Yes, but do you actually work there or do you daydream and so waste precious study time? Do you jump around looking for endless reams of information – oh, just in case, just to make sure? You do? Then change your place of study because this clearly isn't working for you! It helps to find a space where you're less distracted and more focused; your production output increases, results improve and your self-esteem rises. Take ownership, make the change!

STEP 4: MAKING THE CHANGE

Change is always a good thing, although we don't necessarily always think that; it scares us. We like what we do, we're comfortable with our lifelong friend, procrastination. So why change? Well, procrastination affects our performance and our progress (Ackerman and Gross 2005), so changing is a must, especially if we want to:

- do well while on placements
- turn a good grade into an excellent one
- show others we're serious about following this professional route
- enjoy and enhance our learning and practical training
- become less fearful or anxious about our abilities to perform well
- feel and appear more confident in how we present ourselves to peers and patients alike
- grow as a person
- develop as a safe and professional practitioner.

Don't get me wrong, changing a lifelong habit won't happen overnight; it takes time working hard on specific strategies; there's a lot of commitment involved in battling through the many trials and errors until we feel we get it right (Pychyl 2013). But one thing is certain, change won't happen unless we step out and try. Only you can do this; it's your responsibility. So stop dilly-dallying, make a start, define what you want to achieve and what you'll do to get there.

ACTIVITY 4.7   TRIAGE YOUR TASKS

The choice is made but you still need a little help to see the bigger picture and keep on track. You sometimes triage your patients, so why not triage your tasks and duties; prioritise, categorise and move forward.

	DO	DONE
Emergency – attend to that day		
Waiting area – attend to within the week		
Just added to the list – can wait until next week		

You regularly check on your patients once triaged do you not? Then check on your own tasks so you see things moving along and when progress is made. Don't forget to move things up the system so that the 'just added' becomes 'waiting area' and so finally 'emergency'. Still getting stuck a little? Then revisit your learning style and your defining goals (Chapter 1).

Step back and reflect – if my friend needed help with this, what advice would I give? Now take the same advice and stop delaying the reframing process and ultimately the obvious! Don't force the change though; let it happen so it feels more natural. Start with no more than three, small, 10-minute, manageable, achievable tasks per day. Feel you're doing well? Then give yourself a little reward; something you enjoy – movie night, your favourite chocolate!

STEP 5: REVIEWING THE CHANGE

Naming the change forces us out of our comfort zone and into the unknown, but has it worked? Did we get a new perspective on our study, our practice, on ourselves even? Have you experienced a new-found motivation to work between classroom and placement in a more positive, manageable and productive way? So how do you actually feel?

Do you feel more confident in:

* your learning and your practice?
* asking your tutor or placement mentor when you don't know or understand something?
* understanding the 'why' behind the way you learn – theory plus practice?

Does this 'I can do this' attitude shine through in your communication with peers and patients alike?

So to change or not to change, how will you know? You'll never really understand the changes in your procrastination temperature until you see where you've come from and where you're at now:

* a high temperature = procrastination was your best friend
* a low temperature = you've finally shaken if off; your new best friend is 'change and progress' and you've achieved two things:
    o lower stress levels, and
    o changes made, you're more relaxed in your learning.

⚠ **ACTIVITY 4.8　BUDDY BILLBOARDING AND FINAL TEMPERATURE GAUGE**

How much movement has there been in your Buddy Billboarding and procrastination temperature?
　Questions to ask and place on Buddy.

- Where was I going wrong?
- What did I learn in order to change?
- What more can I improve on?
- Is there anything I can still do differently?
- How does this make me feel?
- Has it changed my approach to managing study and practice?

Can you now honestly say that you're well on the way to dumping the negative energy that surrounds procrastination, to breaking the mould and actually enjoying what you're doing? Happy?

TOP TIPS

- ✔ Use a whiteboard to organise your work and your time.
- ✔ Make a note of your procrastinator type.
- ✔ Acknowledge this and identify your goals to move forward.
- ✔ Be honest with yourself.
- ✔ Look at the small steps you can change and jot them down on post-its.
- ✔ Share your experience with a friend and get fresh ideas.
- ✔ Attend procrastination workshops or counselling to work through those guilty or perfectionist feelings.
- ✔ Understand the task set and the learning outcomes – ask if you don't!
- ✔ Look at the bigger picture and identify the smaller parts that make up tasks.
- ✔ Triage your tasks.
- ✔ Learn to delegate family tasks and say 'no' to unreasonable demands so you can manage your workload free from distractions.
- ✔ Tackle one small change at a time and reward your progress.
- ✔ Frequently practise that change until you feel you've mastered it and it's become part of you.
- ✔ Take regular breaks to relax, unwind and re-energise yourself.
- ✔ Frequently reflect on your current practice, review your progress and identify new areas where you can improve.

(Continued)

(Continued)

- ✓ Frequently gauge your procrastination temperature, and note any change.
- ✓ Use your Buddy Billboard often to see what you've still to work on.
- ✓ Make pocket-size positive slogan cards.
- ✓ Change your thinking-and-doing pattern to change your procrastination pattern.
- ✓ Be persistent in your efforts!
- ✓ Find your flow, let procrastination go!

So those are the tips, but don't forget your toolkit at the end of the book!

FURTHER READING

Zen Habits: 'Beating the fears that cause procrastination': http://zenhabits.net/procrastination-fears/

Perry, A. (2003) *The Little Book of Procrastination: How to Stop Putting Things Off.* Suffolk: Worth Publishing.

The Cambridge Student (2016) 'Procrastination: peril of the perfectionist': www.tcs.cam.ac.uk/features/0033285-procrastination-peril-of-the-perfectionist.html

Steel, P. (2011) *The Procrastination Equation: How to Stop Putting Things Off and Start Getting Stuff Done.* Harlow: Pearson Education Limited.

The University of Manchester Counselling Service (2016): www.counsellingservice.manchester.ac.uk/procrastination/

5 EVIDENCE-BASED PRACTICE

⟹ Evidence-based practice – its purpose and benefits
⟹ Improving the quality of care through evidence-based practice
⟹ Researching to identify the latest evidence
⟹ Developing your critical thinking and critiquing skills
⟹ Evidence, clinical reasoning and decision-making
⟹ Using evidence to inform best practice

 CHAPTER OVERVIEW

This chapter looks at the evidence or research that the two professions – nursing and midwifery – draw on to inform and improve practice. It starts by explaining the purpose and benefits of evidence-based practice, exploring how care can be improved through research, and identifying where to find the latest evidence. Once you've found some research, it helps you to read, understand and determine whether it's reliable and credible, and what its strengths and limitations are by applying some critical thinking. The chapter also considers some of the so-called critiquing tools that will help develop your critiquing skills, and concludes by looking at clinical reasoning and decision-making skills to see how evidence can be used to inform your practice.

- Evidence-based practice – its purpose and benefits
- Improving the quality of care through evidence-based practice
- Researching to identify the latest evidence
- Developing your critical thinking and critiquing skills
- Evidence, clinical reasoning and decision-making
- Using evidence to inform best practice
- Top tips

EVIDENCE-BASED PRACTICE – ITS PURPOSE AND BENEFITS

I bet you seek out and use evidence in your everyday lives without really thinking about it. Have you ever looked on popular websites and reviewed a hotel, restaurant, place, or activity you might want to stay at, eat at, go to, or participate in before you decide to book? Have these reviews ever influenced your decisions? Or perhaps you looked up two recipes online and compared them before deciding which one to follow? How did you decide on one rather than the other; maybe you had all the ingredients for the first recipe or the second used less butter, and so you chose that? Or did university league tables or Unistats influence your course choice? If you've undertaken any of these activities then you've certainly used evidence to inform your decisions in your personal life. Great! So, understanding the place of evidence in informing your practice shouldn't be too difficult then. Okay, let's see how it works.

⚠ ACTIVITY 5.1   EVIDENCE-INFORMED DECISIONS

Take what influenced your university course decision. What was it exactly that helped you arrive at your decision? The Unistats alone? Did you research what the students said about the course; look at current employability records; brainstorm the evidence? What thinking or reasoning skills did you use to brainstorm? Finally, map the evidence and the thinking/reasoning skills so that you can see the bigger picture. Can you now see the key role these play in your decision-making? You can? Good, now let's think about all this in relation to evidence-based practice in nursing and midwifery.

So what exactly is evidence-based practice? Well, it's the systematic search for the current, best available evidence that informs decisions about care (Cluett and Bluff 2006). It's this knowledge that you'll use in your daily practice, whether in conversations with patients about their care options, or in meetings with multidisciplinary teams to plan care. Note the word 'current'; note too that the best available evidence changes over time. What may have been common practice 10 years ago is no longer necessarily the best available evidence today. That said, some evidence from 10 years ago is still valid today; in fact it's been further reinforced, and so is more important now than ever.

So where can I find this evidence? Where does it all come from?

Basically, evidence-based practice looks at research, which involves gathering information to provide answers to questions, and the information gathered depends on the question set (Cluett and Bluff 2006; Parahoo 2014; Polit and Beck 2014). Fundamentally, there are two main approaches to research – quantitative and qualitative. However, there's also the combination of both approaches, the so-called mixed methods.

What's what and which is which?

Well, there's 'quality' about the stories, thoughts or feelings of people in a qualitative study and there's 'quantity' – something you can count or measure – in the quantitative approach.

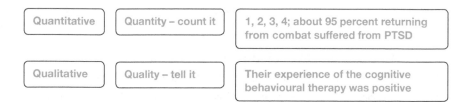

| Quantitative | Quantity – count it | 1, 2, 3, 4; about 95 percent returning from combat suffered from PTSD |
| Qualitative | Quality – tell it | Their experience of the cognitive behavioural therapy was positive |

One method isn't necessarily better than the other. They're simply fundamentally different approaches to gathering information, while the method you use depends very much on what you want to find out and why, and how you intend to use that information.

Research taking a quantitative approach usually uses large numbers of people to measure something, whereas qualitative research generally studies the unique experiences of a small number of people. As an example, let's take the UK census; a UK-wide survey of all people and households on one particular day, undertaken every 10 years. This quantitative measurement of household data started in 1801, with the last data collection in 2011. Each household is asked to complete a questionnaire containing the same questions; so data are collected quantitatively to measure the responses of the entire UK population.

⚠ **ACTIVITY 5.2   QUANTITATIVE DATA SAMPLE**

Check out the 2011 census data on the respective websites of the following agencies and see what information you can glean from these sources; it's amazing what you'll find:

- England and Wales – Office of National Statistics.
- Scotland – National Records of Scotland.
- Northern Ireland – Northern Ireland Statistics and Research Agency.

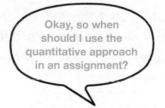

Okay, so when should I use the quantitative approach in an assignment?

If, for example, you're looking for facts and figures to demonstrate that people with learning disabilities have poorer health than their non-disabled peers, then you'd use the quantitative method (Robertson et al. 2010). That's because these studies enable numerical data to be collected about specific areas of interest and allow the researcher to put the results into categories or graphs to make generalisations which relate to the wider population. Think, for example, about research studies that measure things through experiments or closed-question questionnaires, where the results can be applied to the larger population outside of the 'study sample' of participants.

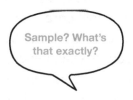

Well, your sample is the number of 'who' you want to target to answer your questions. Let's put it this way – you've the scope, the target sample and of course there's your respondent sample (Table 5.1).

Table 5.1   Scope, target and respondent sample

Scope	The area of study that will help you achieve the purpose of your research (e.g. learning disabled and non-disabled peers)
Target sample	The number of people you want to question (e.g. 100)
Respondent sample	The actual number who completed your survey (74)

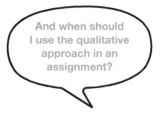

If you want to explore the health and well-being benefits of singing therapy for people with dementia and their carers from a personal experience perspective, then you'd use a qualitative approach (Osman et al. 2014). As you want to gain a deeper understanding of these individuals' unique experiences then the sample doesn't need to be representative. Your sample would be those who've actually experienced what you specifically want to study. Here, you can't make generalisations. But that doesn't mean your findings won't contribute just as much to evidence-based practice.

So there you have it – quantitative and qualitative – sometimes used alone, sometimes together, such as in a mixed methods study about women's decision-making around their choice of birth technique (Kingdon et al. 2009). And then there's the relatively new kid on the block in healthcare research – autoethnography. A strange word, don't you think? Don't be put off though – in real terms, it just means you're examining your professional self in relation to a wider cultural professional context. Actually, you've been using the basic approach from this method since day one of your learning – reflective practice. Yes, reflection! A study on becoming a mother and learning to breastfeed is a good example of autoethnography (Haugh 2016). So, what's the benefit of evidence-based practice?

The Department of Health (DH 2013) identifies three specific benefits of using this type of research in nursing and midwifery:

- It ensures the delivery of best practice.
- It provides value for money.
- It supports the delivery of high quality care.

So let's consider each of these benefits.

The National Institute for Health and Care Excellence (NICE) (www.nice.org.uk/) and the Scottish Intercollegiate Guidelines Network (SIGN) (www.sign.ac.uk/) publish guidelines on how to care for people with a range of conditions, based on the best available evidence. These guidelines form the basis of effective current care in the UK, and are regularly reviewed and updated when significant new findings are published.

⚓ ACTIVITY 5.3   LINKING NICE OR SIGN WITH PRACTICE

So let's check out NICE publications or SIGN guidelines. Access one or other of the websites and see how easy it is to find two or three areas of care that interest you. With regularly published new or updated quality standards, procedures or clinical guidelines you'll surely find something relevant to your field of practice or next placement. So what will it be – long-term conditions, children and young people's care, mental health, maternal health, ear nose and throat conditions, blood disorders?

There are also financial benefits to using evidence-based practice. You can't have failed to read newspaper headlines about the NHS being under increasing pressure to make efficiency savings. Using research to help reduce costs is necessary with our ageing population, limited resources and ever-increasing number of people using the NHS. One of these recently published NICE guidelines shows how cost savings can be calculated through practice, based upon research findings (see Activity 5.4).

⚠ ACTIVITY 5.4   KEY EVIDENCE

Read the NICE Antenatal care guidance updated in March 2016. While most of the guidance hasn't changed since it was last reviewed in February 2014, one part of the evidence base has to reflect research in another area. NICE (2014) now recommend increased uptake of vitamin D supplementation to prevent vitamin D deficiency in pregnant and breastfeeding women, especially pregnant and breastfeeding teenagers. The findings show that vitamin D supplementation costs less than the treatment of its deficiency, thus supplementation is more cost-effective. By following the website links, can you see how they considered this economic evaluation? What evidence was used to make this recommendation?

Drawing on other studies, NICE recommend that vitamin D supplementation is also recommended for other groups whose skin isn't exposed to the sun – children under five, adults over 65, or those with darker skin tones. The combination of research studies used in this latest guidance shows how evidence-based research across diverse healthcare settings can work together for the common good, to improve patient care and service delivery.

IMPROVING THE QUALITY OF CARE THROUGH EVIDENCE-BASED PRACTICE

Florence Nightingale's observations in the 1840s improved the quality of care for patients. She noted the importance of observations and sanitation, and reduced the death rate for soldiers in hospital at that time by improving her practice. Of course, a lot has changed since then, but her observations have contributed to raising the standard of nursing. Now this is your responsibility; you're our 21st-century Florence Nightingale! You've chosen a profession where you're expected to use up-to-date knowledge and evidence both as a student (NMC 2009; 2010) and once fully qualified (NMC 2015a). The Code (NMC 2015a:7) clearly states:

> Always practise in line with the best available evidence. To achieve this, you must make sure that any information or advice given is evidence-based, including information relating to using any healthcare products or services.

This is non-negotiable. You'll learn about evidence-based practice in university and you'll see it in action in your practice learning placement. Just as Nightingale noted, you'll also undertake simple but highly effective activities to prevent the spread of infection:

- washing your hands between patients and between activities with patients, particularly after you've provided personal care and before serving food
- undertaking observations to assess the condition of your client and to alert others if they're deteriorating.

Such action saves lives and improves the quality of care patients receive.

While handwashing and undertaking observations are two areas of nursing and midwifery care that have been researched extensively over time, most studies on these topics are quantitative. If we consider the topics we can understand why this might be so. The research will have used large numbers of the population to show that these activities are necessary. The term you'll sometimes see in quantitative research articles is 'statistically significant', meaning the results of the study couldn't have happened by chance. So research which shows that increased handwashing results in fewer hospital-acquired infections isn't coincidental; it comes from measuring enough people to know that the two are interrelated. Okay, that's the quantitative research, what about qualitative? How does that inform our practice?

Qualitative research draws on studying people, and so nurses and midwives draw on people's experiences to inform how they understand their patients and what might matter to them. While patients want to be safe in hospital, with you washing your hands and undertaking observations, they also want to feel cared for, listened to and respected. It's interpreting these aspects of care that qualitative research addresses. What does it mean to feel cared for? How can professionals listen to and really hear their patients' wishes? How does respect improve care? Well, in a nutshell, it all rests on person-centred care. Want to learn more about this from individuals with long-term conditions? Then complete the following activity.

⚠ ACTIVITY 5.5   PERSON-CENTRED CARE

Click on the link or search for 'patient voices' on a reputable website such as the NHS and listen to patients' views and identify the key points of person-centred care – see e.g. The Health Foundation www. health.org.uk/node/229

Identified and noted? Now in a group with your peers, discuss your findings and map out ways to improve the quality of patient care in your next placement.

RESEARCHING TO IDENTIFY THE LATEST EVIDENCE

How do you find the latest evidence? I guess the most obvious place to start searching for hot-off-the-press evidence is your university library – healthcare databases or the NHS Open

Athens account. It takes time to master the skill of searching for literature; don't let the 'novice frustration' get hold of you! This is where your subject librarian comes in handy. Ask for some training in using the search engines; after all it's their job!

Of course, you can always use elements of your research question to help you search the electronic databases. For example, suppose you want to know how best to care for someone with cystic fibrosis (CF) and you'd like to test out a search? Then, using 'cystic fibrosis' and 'care' as your key search words, complete Activity 5.6.

ACTIVITY 5.6   SEARCHING THE ENGINES

Type 'cystic fibrosis' and 'care' into your university database or Google Scholar if you don't have database access; avoid using non-academic sites such as Google and Wikipedia. So what does your search give you? Hundreds of hits! In that case, the question is too broad, so you'll have to be more specific. So is it the care of babies, children or adults with CF? Which particular aspect of care are you thinking of – physiotherapy, psychological care, diet, or something else? Narrow the focus and structure your search by using the quantitative research question acronym – PICO (Population, Intervention, Comparison and Outcome). For more qualitative research, the acronym PEO (Population, Experience and Outcome) may be more suitable.

Using your cystic fibrosis example, you'll soon see how the two searches take you along different paths to whichever type of evidence you're aiming to uncover. Check out the following example, which uses 'teenagers with CF who require physiotherapy' as a search topic:

PICO – quantitative (heading)	PEO – qualitative (heading)
Population – teenagers with cystic fibrosis	Population – teenagers with cystic fibrosis
Intervention – chest physiotherapy	Experience – chest physiotherapy
Comparison – no physiotherapy	Outcome – feelings
Outcome – effect on chest infections	

While you can see that the two populations are the same with both searches looking at physiotherapy as a focus, only the first has a comparison and measures the differences between two types of intervention. This produces quantitative results – that is, it will compare the effects on chest infections of having physiotherapy as opposed to not having physiotherapy. The second search, on the other hand, talks about the experience of undergoing chest physiotherapy from the teenagers' point of view and documents their feelings about it. This will produce qualitative results.

Depending on where you're at in your education, you may be searching the literature for one or two articles on a topic for an assignment, carrying out an annotated bibliography (AB), or you might want to inform your practice. Alternatively, you may be under- taking your dissertation – a longer piece of work. Regardless, you need to be systematic in your searching. Why not improve the accuracy of your search with Boolean logic or operators – those small words like 'and', 'not' and 'or' (Polit and Beck 2014). Use these and you'll find they come up in the title or abstract. If some- thing keeps coming up in your search that's not relevant, then exclude these articles by adding 'not' to the search. It takes time to learn the process. Again, remember the subject librarian!

DEVELOPING YOUR CRITICAL THINKING AND CRITIQUING SKILLS

When you've found a research article you'll of course read it. But don't just read it as you would an enjoyable, relaxing novel; learn to develop your critical thinking and critiquing skills. Don't assume that:

because it's printed you need to completely agree with it	you can't argue against it and give your own opinion
because the article's author is a well-known researcher, you can't question their findings or methodology	you can't have a view and debate it

So learn to think about what you're reading; ask:

- Does the information sound reasonable?
- Is that logical?
- Do I understand how this research was conducted?

These questions, while hard at first, will help you think critically about the research. Don't be surprised though if you need to read articles two or three times to understand why you need to ask these questions. That's not so unusual – it's all part of the learning process, and, trust me, we've all been there. Don't be surprised either when you see something new or interesting each time you read your research article. Once you've a fairly good grasp of the meaning of the research, you should be able to take your critical thinking to the next level. How exactly?

Well, why not use a critiquing tool to help you achieve a more struc-tured critique of the research article? Sounds good but where can I find these? A few places actually – from online to research textbooks, you're sure to find information and tools to suit your purpose; but why not start with the Critical Appraisal Skills Programme (CASP) which contains critiquing tools for eight different types of research.

So how does this work exactly? Well, the critiquing tool asks specific questions about the research, often presented as two different sets of questions – one for qualitative research and another for quantitative. While this may seem like hard work and time-consuming, with all that backwards and forwards between the research, the textbooks and a research dictionary, it will all pay off – trust me. Your research understanding will be reinforced, you'll know whether the research was conducted well and what its limitations are. Remember, no research is perfect; you'll find strengths and limitations in all research but with well-practised crit-ical thinking skills you'll easily identify these. Oh, and you'll need to report on these!

You might prefer to use a critiquing tool that's specific to the methodology used in the research.

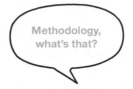

Well, basically it's a way of describing how the research was conducted. When you're critiquing a piece of research it's really important to report on the 'methods' the researcher used – to identify if they were appropriate for the study itself, followed research practice guidance, and produced results which were reliable. Depending on the focus of your own research, you'll have lots of different research methods to choose from – those interesting 'what', 'when' and 'how' processes you'll learn more about as you progress in your studies.

EVIDENCE, CLINICAL REASONING AND DECISION-MAKING

So now you've read the research evidence, what do you do with all that knowledge? Basically, you'll need to think about how that evidence might be used in clinical practice; that's where clinical reasoning skills come into play.

Clinical reasoning is where you gather information, understand the patient or situation, think through their problem, offer choices, evaluate the outcome, or reflect on the clinical experience so you learn from the process. In practice, it fundamentally moves through a five-step process (Table 5.2).

You'll see from this process that it's not just the evidence that informs your decision-making but also the patient's wishes, concerns and other related factors that might affect their care choices.

How does it work? Let's look at how we can apply clinical reasoning to help make decisions in practice. When you worked with your mentor you'll have noticed a situation when they went to care for a patient, immediately knew they were deteriorating, and called for help. Or again, times when your mentor seemed to know exactly

Table 5.2 The five-step clinical reasoning process

1. Consider your patient – their situation, preferences and care needs.
2. Gather information from multiple sources – handover, notes, the patient's condition while taking their observations – consider what's normal and abnormal, and discern relevant information to inform your thinking.
3. Think through their problem – your knowledge of the physiology of their care, the drugs they take, etc.
4. Offer your patient choices based on the information you've gathered in steps 1–3; this allows them to decide what's important to them. Once they've decided, you can evaluate the situation again and see whether the course of action resolved the situation. This may be a temporary or more permanent solution, or you may need to offer other solutions.
5. Evaluate the outcome; reflect on the experience so you can consider how to improve your future practice.

what to say to a relative who was upset. The experienced nurse or midwife will have drawn on both evidence and experience to process the information and/or situation in front of them, and initiate appropriate care. Automatic and intuitive – will I ever get to that stage, I hear you ask? Sure you will: with some 'know-how', some practice and sound clinical reasoning, you'll also instinctively know how to care for your patients to provide the best possible care.

USING EVIDENCE TO INFORM BEST PRACTICE

Remember the NICE/SIGN guidance? Well, much of the 'what you'll do in clinical practice' comes from these sources. You'll see as you read more guidelines that NICE/SIGN search the literature to find research on the topic, and then evaluate the quality of the research to make recommendations. The process is similar to how you'll search, find and critique literature – NICE categorises research on a scale of 1–4 depending on how rigorous the research is.

While the majority of evidence used in the NICE guidance is of a quantitative nature, qualitative research evidence is also pivotal to informing nursing and midwifery practice. Both research methods are used by SIGN. Quantitative research can tell us what we should do, while qualitative is more about the 'how' or 'why' we should do it. Want to check out some research and health reviews to help you understand a little better? Then check online for the Cochrane Library and Evidently Cochrane.

⚠️ **ACTIVITY 5.7   WEAK, STRONG EVIDENCE – NOTE THE DIFFERENCE**

Let's look again at the forms of evidence used in the vitamin D supplementation guidance (NICE 2014). Note that while most of the evidence is weak, one of the qualitative studies was considered strong. Identify and note the weak and the strong evidence as stated in the review. See the difference?

As so much of what we do in the UK in nursing and midwifery is informed by NICE/SIGN guidance, knowing where this evidence comes from, how to scrutinise, critique and discuss its strengths and limitations, how to evaluate how good it is, and how it informs the care choices we offer our patients is an important part of your learning and future role. If you know the evidence for a particular form of treatment is considered weak, you'll be able to help your patient decide on an alternative plan that better meets their needs. Be aware though – in meeting your patient's needs you might think you need to trust NICE/SIGN recommendations alone, without bothering to learn too much about the evidence. That's not the case. What about the patient who doesn't want to follow this recommendation, or who's read the latest research on a new drug they think might help them? Remember the needs of your patient, check the evidence, offer them the best care so they can make an informed choice – after all, it's what we're here for!

Of course, evidence-based practice doesn't stop there. Who knows, you may also have the opportunity to undertake some research and contribute to the knowledge-base of nursing or midwifery in your future career. Now that would be impressive!

TOP TIPS

✔ Set up an informal weekly lunchtime journal discussion club with your peers (virtual in a closed Facebook account or physically face-to-face). Ask them to bring along a research article that's inspired them. Broaden your horizons sharing different articles, links and good practice.

✔ Access the following podcasts:

  o http://ebn.bmj.com/site/podcasts/
  o http://jrn.sagepub.com/site/podcast/podcast_dir.xhtml
  o www.midirs.org/podcast/midwifery-podcast-new-students/

✔ Sign up to alerts for research areas you're interested in.
✔ Subscribe to a journal to give you easy access to research in paper form.
✔ Buy a research methods textbook.
✔ Check out and share the latest news and research posted on the RCM and RCN websites.

So those are the tips, but don't forget your toolkit at the end of the book!

FURTHER READING

Beauchamp, T.L. and Childress, J.F. (2013) *Principles of Biomedical Ethics*, 7th edition. Oxford: Oxford University Press.

Hendrick, J. (2004) *Law and Ethics: Foundations in Nursing and Healthcare*. Chapter 1: 'Law and Ethics', pp. 1–22. Cheltenham: Nelson Thornes Ltd.

Johnstone, M.J. (2016) *Bioethics: A Nursing Perspective*, 6th edition. SW Australia: Elsevier.

Rees, C. (2011) *Introduction to Research for Midwives*, 3rd edition. Edinburgh: Churchill Livingstone, Elsevier.

Saks, M. and Allsop, J. (2012) *Researching Health: Qualitative, Quantitative and Mixed Methods*, 2nd edition. London: Sage.

Schneider, Z. et al. (2012) *Nursing and Midwifery Research: Methods and Appraisal for Evidence-based Practice*, 4th edition. London: Mosby.

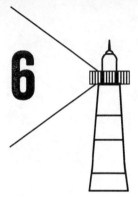

6

SUCCEEDING AT ASSESSMENTS

- Keeping your finger on the pulse – staying on task
- Achieving learning outcomes
- Making and taking notes
- Referencing
- Plagiarism
- Self-directed study
- Continuous assessment
- Oral presentations
- Making it all add up – numeracy and drug calculations
- Timed exams
- Practical clinical skills
- Practice learning placement
- Making the most of your university and practice learning placement feedback

 CHAPTER OVERVIEW

This chapter takes you through the various assessments you'll work through on your nursing or midwifery programme. From the note-making/note-taking process through to referencing, plagiarism, oral presentations, continuous assessment and timed exams, practice learning placements, feedback and self-directed learning, this chapter's assessment-based processes and practical study strategies should help you stay on task. If you understand what's expected in your assignments, you'll soon achieve your learning outcomes and confidently move forward in your professional journey.

(Continued)

(Continued)

- Keeping your finger on the pulse – staying on task
- Achieving learning outcomes
- Making and taking notes
- Referencing
- Plagiarism
- Self-directed study
- Continuous assessment

  o Essays
  o Portfolios
  o Annotated bibliography
  o Critiquing

- Oral presentations

  o From planning to making the message memorable
  o Dealing with difficult situations
  o Stress
  o Presenter's block
  o Technology breakdown
  o Disengaged audience

- Making it all add up – numeracy and drug calculation
- Timed exams

  o Essay-type exams
  o Multiple choice questions
  o Short answer
  o Online

- Practical clinical skills
- Practice learning placement

  o Placement competency booklets
  o Keeping records and handover

- Making the most of your university and practice learning placement feedback
- Top tips

Nowadays, university assignments are a long way from the traditional essays and timed exams only system. While the principle of 'learning outcomes' remains firmly rooted in higher education, the way you're assessed is becoming more varied, more interesting, and more engaging for today's student population. Oh, and more fun to learn! In nursing and midwifery, you're assessed in a variety of ways that makes your learning, understanding and doing more meaningful in the real-life situations you'll face on practice learning placement. Following the requirements of the NMC (2009; 2010), your theoretical knowledge is normally assessed at the end of each trimester/semester/term (according to your university's academic year breakdown), whereas your clinical knowledge is examined as an ongoing activity through achievement of competencies in your placement area, with your progress recorded in your Ongoing Achievement Record (OAR).

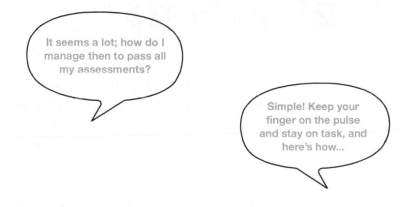

KEEPING YOUR FINGER ON THE PULSE – STAYING ON TASK

With the combination of lectures, practical learning placements and other university commitments, alongside family and social life, it's vital you keep your finger on the pulse and stay on task. Don't do that and you'll find you're constantly chasing yourself, maybe even constantly stressed, and with that your learning process is disturbed. You didn't quite understand, you're not quite sure, you're too tired to think right now, oh, you'll get back to it tomorrow, tomorrow never comes and you lose sight of what you're doing. Don't let this be you!

Planning is easy; sticking to it is harder. So try something different –
reverse planning:

- Note your submission date to your assignment start date – how
  many weeks?
- From writing to researching to planning to unpacking the
  assignment task – set deadlines for each.
- Conclusion to introduction – cross reference connections, check.

So let's get planning so we meet our targets.

> ### ⚓ ACTIVITY 6.1   REVERSE PLANNING – FORWARD THINKING
>
> - You've been given an assignment; what's the submission date?
>   Note it!
> - How many weeks do you have to work on this? Note it!

So how do you plan to move forward to complete your assignment
and meet the deadline? What needs to be done by which target date?
For example, by week six you want to start writing your assignment.
Correct? Then you'll need to have gathered your resources and applied
some critical thinking within those first five weeks. Next, decide how
many weeks you want to spend finding information, and how many
analysing and evaluating what you find? Now work out your reverse
planning target dates. Done that? A tip – keep your eye on the forward
working process and the deadline outcome will be likely, and because
we want you to manage, here's a sample plan to help:

Weeks 1–3:	Unpack the assignment task, start resourcing information, read and make notes, plan your assignment structure
Weeks 3–5:	Critically evaluate, separate what you'll use in your discussion and what you'll discard
Weeks 6–8:	Write up your assignment
Week 9:	Submit assignment

If you're using a proofreader, build in time for submission, feedback and corrections.

Oh, and don't forget your placement travel time and commitments; they're important too!

Well, that's the organisation and planning, now to make the most of it so you stay on task.

A question – so how do you learn best? Remember Chapter 1 where you identified that one main thing that makes learning work for you (http://vark-learn.com); helps you know your stuff, makes the information stick, shows what you've still to learn and, most importantly, helps you remember so you can demonstrate your knowledge in exams and in practice learning placement? Learning style – yes, it's yours so stick to it and use it as only you know how!

That's the organisation, planning, learning style – anything else? Oh yes! Feel you're becoming unstuck? Then refer to your Student Support First Aider (SSFA; Chapter 2), identify the support service you need and arrange an appointment, let someone know, ask for help, accept the help and get back on track with some new-found motivation – keep that finger on the pulse and achieve your learning outcomes.

ACHIEVING LEARNING OUTCOMES

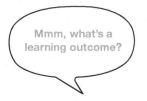

Mmm, what's a learning outcome?

Well, we're teaching you, you're learning from us, and with that we both have expectations on this nursing or midwifery programme. You expect to be able to understand the theory and skills of nursing and midwifery so you successfully pass each module. And as you pass each module, you expect your knowledge to grow and your skills to develop so your practice learning placements are also successful. Correct? That's you, this is us.

A learning outcome is assigned to each individual module, whether theoretical or practical, with first year outcomes being easier than those in second or third year, understandably so. We don't expect you to know everything at once. You can't – why else would you be here learning? We pace your learning, outlining what we expect you to know, understand or be able to do at the end of each module. Take note though – learning outcomes in your nursing or midwifery programme are unlike any other at university. They need to underpin key aspects of clinical practice, and meet the NMC standards and requirements (NMC 2009; 2010). Essentially, you need to achieve and be sufficiently proficient at key points in your learning, so we're confident that you've acquired the knowledge and skills necessary to safely and professionally practise as a nurse or midwife – that's a learning outcome!

> How do I know I've achieved that learning outcome?

Oh, that's easy. It's a demanding programme where you're constantly assessed and your competency evaluated. Fail to meet a learning outcome and we'll tell you, you can be sure of that. Don't forget, we're preparing you so you can meet the NMC standards (2009; 2010) and practise as a safe nurse or midwife delivering safe patient care. So take responsibility for your learning, achieve your learning outcomes, and see graduation day grow ever nearer and professional registration become a reality.

MAKING AND TAKING NOTES

Making notes, taking notes – the same, only different! One we make from information we read when researching and studying, the other from information we hear in lectures, tutorials, workshops. Notes connect our thinking and our learning. We connect old knowledge with new and so we build up our knowledge bank to help us do well in exams and assignments (Weimer 2013). So, how to get the most out of your notes:

1. *Connecting before lectures:* Do you have access to lecture notes in advance? Do you know the topic being covered? If not, read up on it beforehand. Use your Note Nuggets (Figure 6.1) to highlight key points, important dates, names, concepts, theories or practices, make a note of any questions you'd like to ask.
2. *Connecting after lectures:* Remember your notes are the 'skeleton' of your knowledge. It's your responsibility to add the 'meat' of your learning through your research, evidence-based practice and self-directed study (O'Shea 2003; El-Gilany and Abusaad 2012). So, practise building and developing your notes, your before and after lecture connections and you'll surely manage exams, assignments and practice learning placements to achieve your learning outcomes.
3. *What about during lectures?* Again, use your Note Nuggets to jot down key information; number and colour code them so they relate to key points in your lecture handout. Don't try to write down every word; it just won't work.

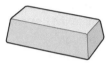

Figure 6.1   Note Nuggets

What about making notes? The tip here is to note the references – the sources you're citing and write any comments in your own words (see referencing and plagiarism sections below). Then make the connections with your lectures, assignment topic or module theme. Connections work!

REFERENCING

Referencing – the very thing we love to hate! Why, oh why, is it so hard? No matter how hard we try, we never seem to get it right. We get mixed up with in-text referencing and end of assignment referencing. Even following the referencing method (http://libweb. anglia.ac.uk/referencing/harvard.htm or www.ukessays.com) step by step, we'll miss out that vital full stop or comma, and then it's comments and lost marks. So is there a method in the referencing madness?

Sure, it's easy really and the latest technology on the market has made it even easier. Check it out for yourself – 'citethisforme' (www. citethisforme.com/), 'EndNote' (http://endnote.com/) and 'refme' (www.refme.com/). Need some help to manage the referencing process? Then check out Table 6.1, which shows the Managing, Recording, Thinking, Referencing system (MRTR) (Gribben 2012). Whatever you do make sure you get it right – always check

Table 6.1   MRTR

Managing:	Organise what and where you search.
	Keep an overview of what you source.
	Plan your time – for reading, thinking, considering, writing up.
Recording:	Alphabetically list the information you want to use.
	Accurately note sources as you go along.
	Make oral summaries using a recording device.
Thinking:	Think things through.
	Critically analyse what you've read to see where it fits with your own thinking and discussion
Referencing:	Reference sources accurately down to the final full stop.
	Check in-text citations, quotations, bibliography and all other referencing levels.

the referencing style you're adopting is in line with the university's referencing policy. And if your university uses the EndNote tool then stick to this; there's no point in confusing yourself trying to learn too many different referencing tools when one can sort it for you.

With a know-how of referencing, you'll surely avoid plagiarism.

PLAGIARISM

Don't do it! Don't plagiarise! It just won't work, you'll get caught and you'll get punished. There's no other way of telling you this. You might call it 'intellectual borrowing' or 'academic clipping' – but me, well, I call it plain old 'pinching'; stealing someone else's work and passing it off as your own (www.plagiarism.org/). Would you like that? No!

Oh, no one will notice, I hear you say. Sure they will. Tutors know their subject area; the discussions in books, articles, the latest evidence-based research (www.nice.org.uk/), who says what, where and why. After all, they've read them too! You're allowed to use authors' work but you must state their name and publication date, and you must write what you've read in your own words! So go on, let me enjoy reading your work, seeing where you've considered the viewpoints, formulated your own opinions, debated, discussed, understood and arrived at a conclusion. Let me know it's yours, not someone else's.

So to keep yourself right – make notes from what you read. Need to copy it word for word so you can think about it later? Then make sure you write 'word for word' or 'direct quote' beside the passage and then re-write the information in your own words once you've processed it all, and come to your own conclusion. If you're including direct quotes, make sure you cite and reference them accurately, otherwise that too is plain and simple plagiarism. And whatever you do, don't sprinkle your work with too many direct quotes; that shows you've read an author's viewpoint but it doesn't mean you've understood it!

So to double-check, always run your assignments through Turnitin (www.turnitinuk.com/) before you're 'turned in' for pinching someone else's work! Yes, keep yourself right! Don't forget that The Code (NMC 2015a) requires you to act with honesty and integrity at all times; this includes academic integrity. Avoid plagiarism and you avoid a professional offence – something that directly brings into question your fitness to practise! Be aware – you can be removed from your programme for plagiarism; it's been known to happen!

SELF-DIRECTED STUDY

> Not quite sure what this is!

Okay, let's simplify it. In a nutshell – you're in the driving seat, taking initiative for and directing your own studies. You're following a specific programme of study, you're given lectures, tutorials, assignments on a variety of topics but how you learn is your responsibility. Tutors can advise, mentors can support, peers can help, but at the end of the day only you can do it. So here are our five pointers:

- Be proactive in your learning.
- Identify your learning needs.
- Use the learning style that works for you.
- Formulate learning goals.
- Do some self-evaluated feedback – learning outcomes met?

Self-directed learning gives you a chance to explore topics and issues in more detail, allowing you to develop specific interests in the area you'd like to work in. With the constantly changing landscape of nursing and midwifery, and the profession's efforts to respond to the demands of an ever-changing society, self-directed learning is the perfect platform for your individual learning; giving you an opportunity to direct your own research through Evidence-based practice (EBP). The first step towards this would be learning how to do an annotated bibliography (AB).

So do you have what it takes to be a self-directed learner (El-Gilany and Abusaad 2012)? Are you self-disciplined, organised, motivated and persistent? Determined to learn, understand, succeed?

Yes! Great! Then you've got what it takes to succeed on your programme. Not quite? Then tap into your SSFA (Chapter 2) and get some key tips on the know-how of self-directed learning.

CONTINUOUS ASSESSMENT

We like, even prefer, this type of assessment; we see how we're doing as we progress through the programme, we build on the feedback and can even see the joined up bits in our learning. It all makes sense. And the best part is we've got lots of time to finish our tasks. Well, not really! Even continuous assessments are timed; there are a limited number of weeks. So remember the reverse planning: get yourself organised, stick to your target dates and you'll enjoy your learning.

ESSAYS

So you've organised your essay timetable, you've unpacked the question and you've done all the research and all the critical thinking and analysis that goes with that (Price and Harrington 2016). Now for the structure – knowing how much to write in each section and what goes where is key to producing a well-structured and well-argued essay.

INTRODUCTION

10% of total word count

What you'll discuss: assignment question re-written in your own words

How you'll go about this: your approach and assignment structure

Your hypothesis: reason for your argument and how you intend to prove your hypothesis is right

How you agree or disagree with the assignment viewpoint

Key concepts relating to the topic

Key points relating to the topic

Explanation or definition of concepts or points

What you'll discuss and why

What you won't discuss and why

Previous relevant research you'll use as evidence

Sometimes an interesting relevant quote

Final sentence leading naturally to the first in the main discussion

MAIN BODY OF DISCUSSION

80% of total word count

First sentence linking from last one in introduction

Main thrust of your argument

A following of the outline presented in your introduction

Your summarised discussion of the topic in sections and sub-sections

One paragraph = one general idea, its purpose and subject matter summarised

Paragraphs relating to your original hypothesis

Body of evidence you discuss, accurately cited and referenced

Information to verify your argument, dates, diagrams, statistics and graphs

For and against examples, evidence, cases, quotations

What you agree with and why   What you don't agree with and why

CONCLUSION

10% of total word count

A logical follow on from the main body of discussion

What you've discussed: how this relates to the original question

Relating clearly back to the introduction

Summary of the main points discussed

Drawing together of all points of your discussion   Summary of your findings

Answer to the discussion's main argument   Your personal viewpoint

How you came to the conclusion you did

Sometimes (if used) the quote included in the introduction to sum up

If appropriate, recommendation for future research or application, but don't include any references – this needs to be a 'summing up' of your work, not the introduction of new ideas!

(Gribben, 2012)

So that's it! Clear enough?

Okay, so I just start with the introduction, finish that, and then move on section by section until I reach the conclusion? Sounds easy enough.

No, don't do that! You'll only feel stuck, unable to move forward, running out of time, and stressed! Work on the sections you find easiest to write, jump around if you need to, and make sure you match up your introduction and conclusion.

So that's the structure, what about language style?

Wouldn't it be simpler if we could write our assignments as we speak? How good would that be – using words we like instead of those unfamiliar words we don't really quite understand? Sorry – you can't!

Learning how to write in an academic-style language takes time but master the skill and you master the academic writing process. Remember, writing in an academic style doesn't mean you've to write in a long-winded, complicated way that's difficult to understand. Want to engage your reader? Then write in a brief, clear, direct, straightforward language style that's readily understood.

Use:

- the third person (he, she, it, they, the writer, the author)
- the active voice, e.g. 'students presented the data'
- the present tense of an author's past reporting, e.g. 'the author recommends'
- academic pointers, e.g. 'as previously mentioned', 'this will be evaluated later in this discussion'.

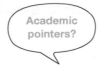

Yes, academic pointers are the cross-referencing connections in your discussion, referring your reader backwards and forwards so they follow the flow of your argument and conclusion.

Don't use:

- the first person (I) unless you're writing a reflective or subjective assignment, or you're instructed to do so
- the passive voice, e.g. 'data were presented by the students'
- contractions of words, e.g. don't, it's, can't
- conversational language, e.g. maybe, really
- figures of speech, e.g. metaphors or hyperboles
- conjunctions at the start of sentences, e.g. because, and, but
- colloquial words or expressions, e.g. sort of, stuff
- two-word verbs when you can use one word, e.g. put off.

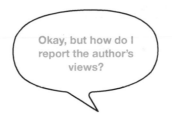

See Table 6.2.

Table 6.2 How to report others' ideas

Use	Rather than
considers or believes	thinks
questions	asks
states or suggests	says
observes	sees
maintains or argues	feels
raises	brings up
appears to be	looks like

Okay that's the language, now for quotations... See Table 6.3.

Table 6.3   Quotations – Dos and Don'ts

Do:

  Use quotations that support your discussion

  Use each quotation appropriately and in context

  Record quotations accurately

  Use 'single' quotation marks when quoting directly

  Use "double" quotation marks when quoting within a quote

  When using a long quotation, use three dots (...) (ellipses) to show that some words have been omitted

  If using part of the original quotation, make sure it makes sense in the context of your own sentence

  If changing words in a quotation to fit the context of your own sentence, put the changed words in brackets [ ]

Don't:

  Use irrelevant quotes

  Use a quotation without commenting on it

  Alter the meaning of a quotation to suit your view

  Use lengthy paragraphs containing irrelevant information as quotations

  Use quotations as padding

Know how to manage all this and you'll develop a robust discussion and avoid plagiarism.

PORTFOLIOS

Keeping a portfolio is part and parcel of your nursing and midwifery life. From student days to professional practice, it's your personal account of the knowledge, skills and professional development you acquire and experience. Look back at your learning so you can move forward to fill the gaps in your development. Remember, portfolios are reflective, subjective – so write in the first person; if you ever let me read it I'd like to know it's your experience not someone else's!

Want to master the art of the professional portfolio from your first practice learning placement? Then follow the advice in Chapter 7 on Reflective Practice and Chapter 12 on Continuing Professional Development (CPD) and you'll surely manage.

ANNOTATED BIBLIOGRAPHY

So what's this all about, I hear you say? What's the ABC of the AB assignment?

Annotate – notes explaining or commenting upon what you've read.

Brief – it's brief, short, concise and to the point.

Critical – it's a critical evaluation of credible, key sources on a specific subject.

So from articles and books, to documents or diagrams, your sources of evidence should include:

- a brief summary of the work's purpose, central themes, arguments, findings and conclusion
- your view of the discussion's strengths and weaknesses
- its relevance to your study and why
- its relationship to other work in the field
- the author's authority in the field
- reliability of the findings and discussion of the author's bias
- the overall impact of the evidence presented on clinical practice or service delivery.

In short, it's a literature review of a selected bibliography focusing on one specific subject.

I don't feel very confident reviewing other people's work. It's difficult knowing how to critically evaluate or even how I should write it.

Just write as you would for essays – follow the academic language style mentioned above. As for critically evaluating – well, you're giving it a close reading, considering the arguments by objectively analysing and evaluating this evidence to help you form your own opinions and conclusions. With some practice, you'll soon know what's expected, and what's more you'll manage. So let's try out a peer exercise; sharing should make it easier.

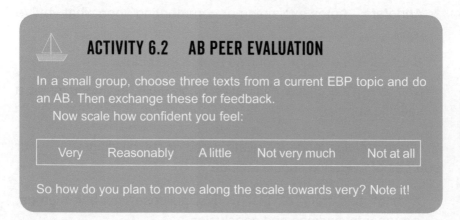

Grasped the ABC of the AB? Great! Understand the process, master the reviewing technique, and you'll come to enjoy the new thinking this brings you.

CRITIQUING

> Critiquing – what's that? Never heard of it – how do I go about this then?

Well in nursing and midwifery studies, you'll be critiquing a lot – comparing and contrasting one article with another. If you're critiquing, you're critically thinking, considering the issue, ana- lysing and weighing up the findings and conclusions (Price and

Harrington 2016). Oh, and in all this you'll be forming your own opinions and drawing your own conclusions about this article and that one. Much like the essay writing style and AB points mentioned above, except a fuller discussion. That's critiquing!

ORAL PRESENTATIONS

We all like to talk; easier in many ways than putting things on paper. So how do we get our message across and show we know what we're talking about?

FROM PLANNING TO MAKING THE MESSAGE MEMORABLE

Simple, get the planning right and you'll get the timing right, and your message should be memorable.

Okay, you've been given the topic, you've researched it, you've pulled out the key information you want to talk about and you've discarded the irrelevant. What next? Two things – from the planning to the newsreel delivery, follow the Presentation Process using your Presentation Pyramid and you're sure to confidently deliver a presentation and message that's memorable.

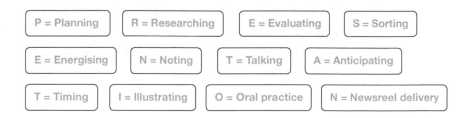

Presentation Pyramid

On a practical level, decide how many slides you'll use to deliver your message; how many bullet points, illustrations, activities, etc.

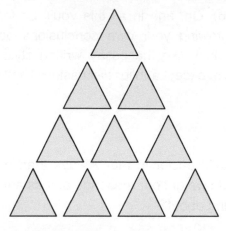

Figure 6.2 Presentation Pyramid

⛵ ACTIVITY 6.3   ACCESSIBLE POWERPOINTS

Want to give your PowerPoints the accessibility factor so no one is excluded? Then test your accessibility knowledge and brainstorm with your peers noting what you consider works well and what doesn't in PowerPoints (Appendix 5).

Two things to keep in mind:

- Anticipate questions – make a note of possible questions and formulate your answers. Do this and you'll feel in command of the message you want to get across.
- Know when to stop taking questions – don't do this and you'll run the risk of that 'forgettable message'.

So start planning, consider all angles and enjoy your newsreel.

DEALING WITH DIFFICULT SITUATIONS

So how do we get through those difficult situations? The unexpected happenings? Simple! Prepare for them; they do happen you know, and knowing how to cope should make your presentation run smoother. Work out a few positive strategies, ask friends for some strategy tips, and practise them.

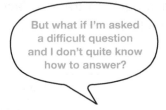

But what if I'm asked a difficult question and I don't quite know how to answer?

There are two ways of dealing with this on the day – say you'll come back to it later once you've thought a little more about it; whatever you do, don't bluff it! Or simply return a difficult question with a question that opens it up to the audience? It works! But whatever you do, remember the presentation key – 'quietly confident'.

STRESS

Stress – that thing we love to hate! It's there – when researching and pulling our ideas together, when thinking about our presentation, and, uhm, dare I say it – even while we're presenting. So how do we put the lid on that unavoidable thing? Basically, organise your stress! Take steps to minimise stress on the day:

- Stress management – attend workshops, learn strategies that work for you.
- Practise your presentation – timing, pace, voice projection, command of information, structure and detail, using technology.

Want to gauge your stress 'temperature'; see how interested your audience could be; how well your strategies are working? Then face the honesty gang – your friends! Practise, feed back and monitor each other's stress. Just bag yourself some self-belief – you're in charge, you can do this!

PRESENTER'S BLOCK

Remember, you're in charge. If you appear positive and assertive, your audience probably won't realise you've gone blank but if you do – take a drink of water, look at your prompt cards, recap the last bullet points and even ask if there are any questions at that point.

This should get things back on track. A few tips for your prompt cards are shown in Table 6.4.

Table 6.4 Accessible prompt cards – Dos and Don'ts

Do:	Don't:
Use clear bullet points	Overload text and references
Give brief additional information	Cram in too many annotations
Use clear highlighting: colours or symbols	Use too many colours or symbols
Match card numbers with PowerPoint slides	Use unnumbered cards

TECHNOLOGY BREAKDOWN

Trust me, it happens – even to those who like technology, and if you don't, it's a disaster on the day.

Always check the technology you're using is working; give it a trial run the evening before and the hour before when you set up. Check it out with a friend and always have a technology specialist on hand to support you if the worst happens and it completely 'crashes'. And trust me, it can 'crash'! Always keep a manual backup so that if worst comes to worst, prompt cards or a PowerPoint hard copy can save the day. Remain confident and focus on the message!

DISENGAGED AUDIENCE

It happens to the best of us. We prepare a well-researched topic and work hard on the presentation – the structure, our presentation skills – so we can get the message across: full of enthusiasm we start presenting and the unexpected happens...

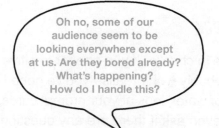

Don't be put off. Do one of two things:

- Questions – they'll quickly become engaged when you ask what they think of specific points you've mentioned so far; or simply ask if they'd like to ask a question at this point, generate discussion to engage the disengaged!
- Focus on the one person who looks interested – look at them, look back at your presentation screen, scan the room confidently and be assertive. Oh, and if you look positive, interesting and enthusiastic, it might just rub off! Okay, sorted? Let's roll!

MAKING IT ALL ADD UP – NUMERACY AND DRUG CALCULATIONS

Numbers – love them, hate them, even phobic about them? You can't avoid them though. So how do we make it all add up in our drug calculations? Practise, practise, practise! Seriously, use strategies and techniques that work for you – BBC bitesize (www.bbc.co.uk/education) or other similar online calculation tools, a pocket calculator, drug calculation tables (www.testandcalc.com/), a calculations manual (Baxter Pharmacy Services 2014), make your own medicine mind map or cut out shapes of tablets and syringes, or how about a part-time job in a pharmacy where seeing the medicine, its shape and size regularly supports your visual learning. Oh, and if you've forgotten the basics of numeracy, then check out a primary maths book (Oxford Dictionaries 2013) – great for revising! So when learning drug calculations, remember the numbers not the words, and chunk your learning for easy recall.

A thing to note – in practice, two people generally check the medication before administration, so knowing you're not alone should lift the pressure of dealing with numbers when you don't like them. And if you're scared or have a phobia, then tap into your SSFA (Chapter 2) and talk to a counsellor. Don't leave it too late or nothing will add up for you.

TIMED EXAMS

ESSAY-TYPE EXAMS

While there's more variety in how we're assessed nowadays, writing an essay in an exam is still part and parcel of the assessment process. It's timed and so is much less detailed than the continuous assessment essay – no need for footnotes, citations, references. But demonstrating your knowledge in a timed essay-type exam requires a certain discipline and technique. You need to know how to get the message across concisely and accurately, how to discuss and debate key points, and how to say the relevant, not the irrelevant. Oh, and when to stop waffling on just to fill up the page. Yes, we know waffling!

We want you to succeed, you want to succeed – so here's the know-how-to-succeed-technique.

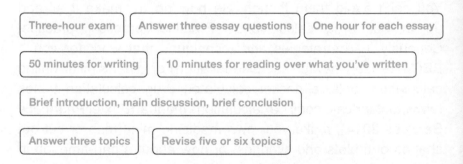

Whatever you do, don't make the mistake of writing a sample essay and learning it off by heart so you can write it in the exam. That just won't work. You're restricting what you can do with that information and I'm not actually seeing what you know. Quite the opposite – I'm seeing what you don't know. Oh, and what definitely won't work is revising three topics only! Yes, you might take the chance and be lucky that those same three topics come up in the exam. Trust me – that might happen once but it certainly won't happen again, so don't risk triggering panic in your exam.

Instead, what you need to trigger is information recall, so highlight key points when practising essay writing. Remember, it's an academic exercise so use academic language style, not chatty language! Want to succeed? Then use past papers to practise and time your essay writing skills using this technique and you're sure to manage.

MULTIPLE CHOICE QUESTIONS (MCQS)

Yes, no, perhaps, maybe, could be, definitely – oh, the confusion! Love them or loathe them, we've still got to do them. The answer's always there, so you'd think multiple choice tests were easy, but well, not always. There's always a spanner in the works that throws doubt on your answer. So how do we work it all out? Simple – spot the spanner, sharpen your decision-making skills and unpack the answer. So here's the method; your five-step answer finder:

Read the question, cover up the answers and try to recall the answer in your head.

Now read all the answers.

Rule in, rule out – look at answers one by one and get rid of the 'Definite no'.

Look for the opposites and rule out the 'Perhaps', if only other things were relevant.

Work out why the spanner is exactly that, and rule it out.

So there you have it – your answer, the 'Definite yes'!

Not practised this enough? Still unsure? Then trust your instinct and guess the most obvious. You never know, you could be right and gain that mark!

Learn your stuff, learn the method and you'll easily master the multiple choice exam.

SHORT ANSWER

It's exactly what it says – short answer. You're asked questions and you're expected to give concise answers only. Write any more than that and you're wasting your time. Oh, it's nice to show that you know your stuff but you won't get any brownie points for writing more than necessary. So 'short' is the answer!

> But how do I know how much to write?

Easy! In short answer question exams, you're given the allocated mark beside the question. This indicates roughly how much you need to write; when two marks are allocated they're only looking for two points, not two paragraphs or two pages. A tip – double up the writing time. Confused? Well, if it's a two mark question then it's worth four minutes of writing, so time yourself.

ONLINE

> Oh, I like online exams.

You're on your own, there's no one else around and you've all the time in the world. Not quite! Sure you'll be on your own in a quiet corner somewhere – at home, office, study room but you don't have all the time in the world. Online exams are generally timed. So don't make the mistake of completing half and thinking you'll finish it later. That won't work as you'll be 'locked out'. So make sure you:

- know how much time the exam takes
- actually have the time to complete the exam from start to finish before logging on and setting the clock running
- tell others you're doing your assessment and can't be disturbed
- put a 'Do not disturb' sign on your door
- switch off all phones, music and other devices
- set your timer and start
- answer the questions in sequence, unless you can scroll up and down answering what you feel is easiest first so you don't feel stuck or stressed.

Oh, and to make the process easier – learn your stuff and know the process for each type of online test, whether it's drug calculations or MCQs. Do that and you'll surely succeed.

PRACTICAL CLINICAL SKILLS

OBJECTIVE STRUCTURED CLINICAL ASSESSMENTS (OSCAs) AND OBJECTIVE STRUCTURED CLINICAL EXAMINATIONS (OSCEs)

So what's this all about and what's the difference? Okay, let me explain: Objective Structured Clinical – A for Assessment and E for Examination, the OSCA is ongoing, the OSCE is the final test; that's the difference. Effectively, it's where your clinical skills are being tested. But what's the set-up?

Your university's clinical skills centre allows you to practise your practical skills, from taking blood pressure to practising injections to reviving a newborn baby, and to do this you move from station to station, timing, talking your way through the process and completing documents. Skills refined, you're ready to demonstrate your professional competency in what could be a real-life situation. So, where you can, learn the processes of each skill and practise with your peers in the simulation clinic; and where you're uncertain practise with your tutor. Practise well in simulation and you'll be fit to practise in real life.

PRACTICE LEARNING PLACEMENT

Your practice learning placement isn't just about putting what we've learned in theory into practice in a real-life clinical situation. Sure, it's that – and more. Working in a real-life environment gives us the unique opportunity to reflect on how we're doing, what we've learned and have still to learn, whether nursing or midwifery is all we expected, and if it's the right profession for us. So how do we keep track of all this?

PLACEMENT COMPETENCY BOOKLETS

Completing your practice placement competency booklet is vital to your progress, whether it's a paper-based copy or an online account of your clinical experiences. It's feedback on how you're doing on each placement, and gives you an overall view of where you started and where you are in your professional learning – that bigger picture. It allows all involved in your professional education – tutor, mentor, you – to evaluate whether you're achieving your NMC (2009; 2010) competencies and are considered fit for practice. It's about proving you can link theory to practice.

Think of your practice placement competency booklet as the start of your professional reflective practice, so use it seriously and be diligent in completing it honestly. Otherwise, it just won't work. Remember, you need to be a safe practitioner – we're giving you the tools, it's your responsibility to use them! Mmm, reflective practice? Don't worry, we'll tell you about all that in Chapter 7. Follow the process while you're a student and you'll follow it for life.

KEEPING RECORDS AND HANDOVER

The Code (NMC 2015a) instructs nurses and midwives to 'work with others to protect and promote the health and wellbeing of those in your care'. So what does that actually mean for record keeping and handovers? For our patients? For us?

We look after our patients, we're with them for a limited time and we've kept track of how they're doing that day – shift over and we hand over their care to someone else, and we go home happy.

Great! We've kept ourselves right, fulfilled our ethical duty of care and we've met the NMC professional practice requirement to keep records up to date and ensure a smooth handover (Scovell 2010). Happy at home with a well-earned cuppa, and suddenly...

> Oh no, I got distracted and forgot to write the day's medical tests update; I did mention them though.

Not good enough, I'm afraid. Forgetting to record that could be a disaster waiting to happen and it goes against The Code! Listen, if it's important enough to be said it's important enough to be written. Don't rely on someone else's memory. Keep your patient safe, keep yourself safe, keep your professional registration safe. Remember, only you can take full responsibility for your actions – don't trust someone else to do it for you!

> But I'm only a student; how do I know what's in a handover?

In a nutshell, a patient's record contains factual information about their care and is a legal document, which can be used in a Court of Law, if necessary. Sure, it tells the 'story' of their care but, whatever you do, don't write it as a story; use the correct terminology, be factual and objective, keep it brief and to the point. Don't worry though, observe your peers and mentor, learn the process and language, try it out, understand what's happening and why, and you'll soon learn on the job. Make your learning easier – devise a visual symbol association system to support information recall for your own personal memory use, e.g. patient's mood = smiley face, sad face; appetite = knife/fork. Oh, and a thing to note – different health boards and universities recommend using different record-keeping processes, such as CHAPS (Clinical picture; History; Assessment; Plan; Sharing of information) (Owen and Candelier 2010) and SBAR (Situation; Background; Assessment; Recommendation) (NHS Institute for Innovation and Improvement 2008).

So keep the process right, keep yourself right – check out yours. Remember, at the end of the day, it's all about patient safety and responding to the needs of your patients and the ever-changing healthcare environment.

MAKING THE MOST OF YOUR UNIVERSITY AND PRACTICE LEARNING PLACEMENT FEEDBACK

We want to know how we're doing; how well we've done on that assignment, how well on our placement. We need to see how our actual performance matches up with the expected learning outcome. Is there anything more we could do to improve what we're doing? Feedback, that's what we need – whether 1:1, online, in small groups or peer feedback, it's a learning opportunity that makes what we do meaningful and valuable in our nursing and midwifery practice (Somerville and Keeling 2004). Oh, but when we get it we find it's a mixed bag – encouraging, upsetting, challenging, engaging, and sometimes even very personal! Well, at least that's how we take it; that unexpected, unwanted 'criticism'.

I don't particularly click with my tutor or mentor, so it feels personal.

Sure it's personal; it's about your work, showing where you've done well or need to improve. It's not meant to give you a hard time. No! Whatever the feedback, it's meant to raise questions, challenge your thinking, enhance your reflection, help you learn better so you understand better, help you link your learning to all future practice, even test your commitment to your nursing or midwifery profession. So whatever you do, don't take it personally – remove the 'person' and keep the 'ally'. Remember, it's what you do with the comments that makes the difference not what's actually said and by whom. Need a helping hand to see the bigger picture and put things in perspective? Then use the feedback CAP

Consider – what's said where and why; what's the 'ally' you'll feed forward

Assess – how you're developing as a learner; reflect on the feedback and how to make the most of the comments

Practise – new strategies and methods that support your learning in class and in placement.

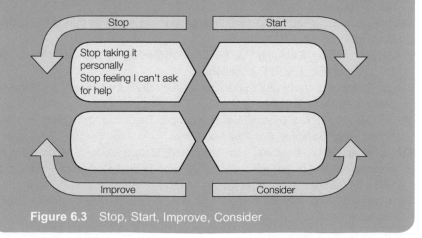

△ ACTIVITY 6.4   STOP, START, IMPROVE, CONSIDER

Reflect on your recent placement experience and your mentor's feedback, both positive and negative. Using the Stop, Start, Improve, Consider technique, note how you intend to use the feedback so you move forward in your learning.

Stop

Stop taking it personally
Stop feeling I can't ask for help

Start

Improve

Consider

Figure 6.3   Stop, Start, Improve, Consider

Do this and your feedback will surely feed forward. Do this and you'll become the knowledgeable and skilful practitioner you set out to become.

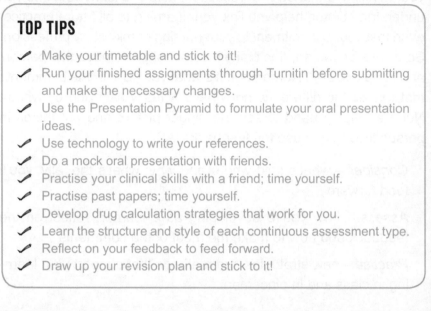

TOP TIPS

- ✓ Make your timetable and stick to it!
- ✓ Run your finished assignments through Turnitin before submitting and make the necessary changes.
- ✓ Use the Presentation Pyramid to formulate your oral presentation ideas.
- ✓ Use technology to write your references.
- ✓ Do a mock oral presentation with friends.
- ✓ Practise your clinical skills with a friend; time yourself.
- ✓ Practise past papers; time yourself.
- ✓ Develop drug calculation strategies that work for you.
- ✓ Learn the structure and style of each continuous assessment type.
- ✓ Reflect on your feedback to feed forward.
- ✓ Draw up your revision plan and stick to it!

So those are the tips, but don't forget your toolkit at the end of the book!

FURTHER READING

UK Essays 'Annotated bibliography': www.ukessays.com/essays/health/annotated-bibliography.php

Duffy, K. (2013) 'Providing constructive feedback to students during mentoring', *Nursing Standard*, 27(31): 50–56.

Hutchfield, K. and Standing, M. (2012) *Succeeding in Essays, Exams and OSCEs*. London: SAGE Publications.

Maslin-Prothero, S. (ed.) (2005) *Bailliere's Study Skills for Nurses and Midwives*. London: Bailliere Tindall.

Roche, M. (2013) *The Sketchmore Handbook*: *The Illustrated Guide to Visual Note Taking*. Berkeley, CA: Peachpit Press.

Tett, L. et al. (2012) 'Learning from feedback? Mature students' experiences of assessment and higher education', *Research in Post-Compulsory Education*, 17(2): 247–260.

Whitehead, E. and Mason, T. (2003) *Study Skills for Nurses*. London: SAGE Publications.

7 REFLECTIVE PRACTICE

⇒ Reflective practice – what is it exactly?
⇒ In-action, on-action reflection – what's the difference?
⇒ The ELG process
⇒ 3Rs – recap, review, reflect
⇒ The reflective practitioner – continuing professional development

---

 CHAPTER OVERVIEW

Using ELG (Experience, Learning, Gaps), this chapter takes you through the different aspects of a learning log and the role of reflection in your learning process. It helps you to understand how to reflect and to develop your reflective practice techniques so you'll confidently complete assignments, manage your practice learning placements and, with that, your professional practice should continue to improve.

- Reflective practice – what is it exactly?
- In-action, on-action reflection – what's the difference?
- The ELG process

  o Experience
  o Learning
  o Gaps

- 3Rs – recap, review, reflect
- The reflective practitioner – continuing professional development
- Top tips

REFLECTIVE PRACTICE – WHAT IS IT EXACTLY?

In everyday life we do, we think and we learn. Simple, we've learned! So I guess we do things better next time around. Maybe so – but what about our nursing or midwifery practice learning placement activities? Is it all really that simple? What is reflection really, what does it all mean and what's the purpose of it all? What's the best way to learn the reflective process so I become good at reflection in my learning and move through the reflective stages from descriptive to analytical to critical? How exactly will it help me as a practitioner and support my revalidation? Okay, lots of questions, so let's see what reflective practice means to you just now – as a student; a budding practitioner. You're a positively curious student willing to learn? Correct? You're aiming to be a knowledgeable, caring, professional practitioner? Correct? And you want to make it all work? Correct? Then let's look at reflective practice and see what it's really all about. Understand all that and it's surely going to work!

In nursing and midwifery, Reid describes reflective practice as 'a process of reviewing an experience of practice in order to describe, analyse, evaluate and inform learning about practice' (1993: 306). The *Oxford Dictionary* describes 'reflection' as 'serious thought or consideration' (http://oxforddictionaries.com/definition/reflection). So take that with you into your practice and you'll learn to think more deeply, widely, broadly and more critically so that all your future practice and learning are 'informed', both as a student and registered practitioner. Yes, you're a lifelong learner in nursing and midwifery – always seeking to improve practice and patient care through reflection and fulfil the NMC (2015c) revalidation requirements. Let's note the process then!

> serious thinking + following process = celebrating what we did well and repeating it, or = doing things differently next time around

> apply theory to practice + practice to more theory = ideal reflector and professional practitioner

But firstly, let's get a few things clear about reflective practice. It's your experience so there's no right or wrong concerning how you feel, what you think, what you learn. It might be similar to how other people experience things but really it's all unique to you. You're 'inside' the situation (subjective), not 'outside' looking on or reading about it (objective) – so remember, if you ever share your journal, the person reading it wants to know it's your experience in that situation – not theirs (see Table 7.1)!

Table 7.1 Reflective journal writing style

Why:	Your experience, your thinking, your learning, your personal perspective
What:	Informal, personal writing style using the first person 'I'
Why:	You're actively learning
What:	Ask questions, consider your thoughts and feelings, relate your ideas to those of others, connect what you've already learned to what you're now discovering in practice, and report using the active voice, e.g. 'Based on my observations, I recommend we use...'
Why:	Past tense (what you know from theory or previous practice)
	Present tense (what you're discovering as reality in your current practice)
	Future tense (what you plan to do in the future to improve your practice)

Okay, Table 7.1 outlines the 'what' and 'why', now for some useful phrases:

I think   I felt   I realised   I felt uncomfortable with   On reflection I now think

Oh, and where appropriate, don't forget to refer to academic texts or professional body directives – that's important too. Right, that's the fundamentals of reflective practice! Want to make the most of putting them into practice? You do? Then firstly let's identify your reflector type. Join that up with your preferred learning style and you'll confidently manage the process.

⛵ ACTIVITY 7.1　YOUR REFLECTOR TYPE

As a curious student and budding practitioner, how do you think just now? How does that differ from what you need to do in reflective practice? Need to change anything? Note it!

Table 7.2　What type of reflector are you?

Type	Description	Tick here
Linker-thinker	I think about what I know and how that ties up with what I'm doing	
'If only' thinker	I think about what I don't know but maybe should know	
Joined-up thinker	I know, think, do, learn, do differently	
Out-of-the-box thinker	I think of different and diverse possibilities to facilitate learning the bigger picture	
Over-thinker	I think too much and then worry about not doing it right	
Critical thinker	I objectively analyse, evaluate and consider	
On foot doer-thinker	I think while I'm doing; why I'm doing it this way and what I need to do differently to improve	
Global thinker	I think about all factors related to tasks and all the learning possibilities	

Well that's reflection but what about in-action and on-action reflection (Schön 1983, 1987 in Johns 2013). What's the difference?

IN-ACTION, ON-ACTION REFLECTION – WHAT'S THE DIFFERENCE?

Well ultimately they achieve the same thing, you just do them at different times – that's the difference.

In-action:

> taps into your working memory; the here and now on-the-spot reflection of your thinking and feeling, where you can log the details as things happen.

Concerned you don't have time? Then create your personal note-taking system to log your reflections; for example, using a blank page notebook where you can use a combination of visual imageries, colours, bullet points, storyboarding, single word descriptors (Somerville and Keeling 2004; Gribben 2012). Build in a few minutes after tasks or during break times, pull out that pocket notebook – record it, reflect, and always remember patient confidentiality – don't name names! Oh, and remember, it's a notebook – your memory jogger for completing your reflective journal – not a novel, so be brief!

On-action:

> relies more on your long-term memory; where you're looking back at what happened that day, forming a retrospective picture of how things went in practice.

Worried you'll forget the detail? Again, pull out that notebook and quickly record as you go along so you can reflect further later. Realistically, how long does it take to jot down a few abbreviations, symbols, details? Short, colourful, visual notes work! Not for you? Then find a way that does and stick with it! Whatever it takes! And remember, even in the briefest of notes on your reflective experience, it's your responsibility to safeguard patient confidentiality at all times (NMC 2015a).

I'm new at all this, so what's the best way to learn reflective practice so I become good at it?

Okay, reflective practice is essentially a thinking process that informs both your learning process and your understanding. It challenges your knowledge, values, behaviours and beliefs (Somerville and Keeling 2004). Throughout your life, you're reflecting on different situations – what happened and why; what if I'd done this and not that, would it have made any difference; maybe if I make one small change next time around things would work out better; okay, I need to learn about that so I'm better prepared if a similar situation happens again – it's all a learning curve, a lifelong learning process. Your nursing and midwifery practice is no different; throughout our career we think and we learn, and we put into practice, and in that we become more confident at what we're doing – quite the expert thinkers and doers (Gopee 2003). By studying how we do things, our thinking and learning helps us to make sense of what has happened. It helps us to feed back so we can feed forward and always improve our way of working. That's the purpose of our reflection – think, learn, improve (www.skillsyouneed.com/ps/reflec tive-practice.html).

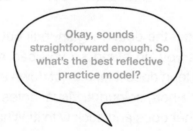

In your nursing and midwifery studies, you'll be expected to use the traditional models of reflection such as Gibbs (2013), Rolfe et al. (2001), Johns (2013) or Taylor (2006) (see Appendix 6) to help you learn the reflective practice process and put theory into practice. There's no right or wrong model, but don't make the mistake of launching straight into your reflective practice without first checking your programme handbook to see if there's a specific model you should use. While some tutors leave you to decide on the model of reflection, others prefer to specify it to help you develop your reflective writing skills from descriptive to critical reflection (Howatson-Jones 2016), so get this verified. Oh, and if there's anything you don't understand about the reflective practice process, just ask! It's best to ask at the outset rather than fumble your way through and lose essential marks at the end.

So take time to learn about the process and how to apply it. Get into the habit of reflection, think about everything you're doing. Don't force it, though; let it happen naturally and reflection will come naturally to you. Be careful not to over-think; do that and you run the risk of becoming anxious, a bit of a perfectionist obsessed with always wanting to get it just right, and so rather than enjoying the learning you get from reflective practice, you'll start to question your own abilities and doubt your capabilities. So what's it to be – a weaker, uncertain practitioner or the stronger, confident one you stepped out as on that first day? Don't worry, visualise confidence and proficiency, stay positive, and watch your self-awareness and learning develop and grow as you prog-ress from the first to the final year. Track the progress from your descriptive portfolio (year one) to the analytical (year two) and the critical (year three).

There are plenty of traditional reflective models in nursing and midwifery; some easier to understand and apply than others, but how about trying out my newly developed evaluative tool – the three-step ELG reflective process? If you think as you do, you'll learn before you do it all again – and most likely even better or differently!

THE ELG PROCESS

Well okay, it's not your traditional reflective practice model, but it marks the three main stages in your reflective practice:

- *Experience* – your personal experience of the practical situation
- *Learning* – what you've learned from your personal experience and how that links with your previous knowledge

- *Gaps* – what you've still to learn from your experience and your mentor's feedback so you can improve your lifelong practice.

So, traditional or not, ELG is designed to help you reflect on your practice so that you become a more engaged student and a better practitioner – and surely that's a good thing! But take note, this isn't just a quick thinking exercise; it's much more than that. Remember, reflection requires commitment and responsibility (Johns 2013) so when you're tired at the end of that long shift, gently remind yourself of the commitment you made when you signed up to the profession and the responsibility that brings to professionally develop your learning and your practice. Then reflect!

So, to use ELG effectively, you'll need to identify and describe the factual and not the hearsay of:

- your placement activities – what happened
- your experience of them – feeling and thinking
- how it went – good, bad, confusing
- any theoretical knowledge you already have that helps you make sense of what happened
- the diverse, positive gifts you bring to your placement
- anything else you could have done differently
- your mentor's feedback and how that helps develop reflection skills, future learning and practice (Johns 2002).

Oh, and don't forget your plan of action for next time around. That's important too!

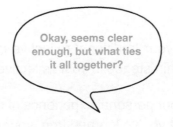

Seriously, in a word, 'reflection' – that's what ties it together. You think about what you do on placement activities then you tie that up with what you've learned in class, from books or journals, as well as through previous experiences and knowledge. Clear enough? Still confused? Then let's get the gist of the ELG process by looking at something fundamentally basic in healthcare – the aseptic technique.

Mosby's Medical Dictionary (2016: 144) describes the aseptic technique as:

> any health care procedure in which added precautions, such as the use of sterile gloves and instruments, are used to prevent contamination of a person, object, or area by microorganisms.

As a key part of the NMC's essential skills cluster required for pre-registration nursing or midwifery (2009; 2010), you'll learn all about this technique in your infection control lectures. It's high on their agenda and should be high on your agenda too! So let's test it out. You're being assessed on the aseptic dressing technique (www.cetl.org.uk/learning/) in clinical skills simulation. You've been taught the three principles:

1. Maintain asepsis.
2. Expose the wound for the minimum time.
3. Employ an efficient procedure.

And the key preparation areas where these apply; prepare the patient, the nurse and the equipment. So you followed the process, completed the task but did you remember to check the comfort of the patient; consult the care plan; clean the trolley surface? Oh, and complete the documentation? Using ELG, let's reflect on your experience.

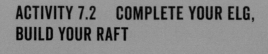

ACTIVITY 7.2   COMPLETE YOUR ELG, BUILD YOUR RAFT

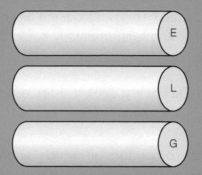

E – What you *experienced* practising the aseptic technique while dressing a wound

L – What you've *learned* from that experience; can you link what you already knew (theory) to your clinical skills simulation experience (practical)?

G – Is there anything you feel you've still to learn (*gaps*) to improve your experience next time around? Or is there anything you feel you did well that you'll continue to practise?

Now transfer your familiar clinical skills simulation reflective experience to the currently non-familiar clinical situation. Feel an example would help you see how reflective learning is transferable from one clinical situation to another, and why infection control is uppermost in practice?

EXPERIENCE

On placement at a large neonatal intensive care unit, I was part of the medical team performing a lumbar puncture on a premature baby, born at 32 weeks gestation due to the mother's pre-eclampsia. I was working under the supervision of my mentor, assisting her and other experienced staff. The baby's observations had changed and there was a concern raised of the potential for septicaemia developing.

Neonatal babies are predisposed to early-onset septicaemia in cases where the mother has group B streptococcus in her gastrointestinal, reproductive or urinary tract (Lee 2014), and so we were assessing the baby's condition through blood tests and by draining cerebrospinal fluid (CSF).

As part of this procedure, I was asked to catch the CSF in a universal container while the needle was in place. I noticed, however, that the doctor had quickly moved from another patient to this one without washing her hands or cleaning the baby's lumbar region before inserting the needle. She'd also touched the universal container, as I tried to hold it higher to catch all the fluid safely. This concerned me, as the reason for carrying out the lumbar puncture was to check for the risk of infection, particularly the early stages of septicaemia, and one of the ways to prevent the spread of this is through proper handwashing by all those coming into contact with the baby (Lee 2014). The RCN (2005) also highlights the importance of minimising the risk of cross-infection through hand hygiene disposable items such as gloves and aprons.

As it was my first time assisting in a lumbar puncture procedure and I was a junior member of the team, I felt I couldn't challenge the doctor about infection control. By the time I gathered the courage to say something, the doctor had moved on to her next patient. We were short staffed that day and she had to cover more patients than normal.

LEARNING

I found this incident extremely challenging and regretted not mentioning infection control before the needle had been inserted into the baby. I decided to talk to my mentor about this situation and asked about the lumbar puncture procedures on neonatal babies at risk of infection. She reminded me of the NMC Code (2015a) covering patient safety and minimising risk for the patient, and my obligation to understand and apply it in practice, even as a student and junior member of the team.

To help me manage future similar situations, we decided I should ask the doctor about normal procedures from their perspective, as a way of helping my learning and developing my interpersonal skills. When I mentioned to the doctor what I'd observed and about my concerns, she was apologetic and thanked me for raising the issue. She acknowledged it was remiss on her part, and that being extra busy shouldn't be a reason for forgetting the importance of infection control. Being able to approach the doctor made me realise that regardless of the seniority levels in the team, we're all equally responsible in our duty of care for our patients' well-being. I also felt it helped my confidence for future practice.

GAPS

On reflection, I realise that my mentor was correct and positive in her feedback, and that not speaking up may have put the baby at risk even more. Being reminded early in my professional development of my duty of care towards the well-being of all patients under my care is a strong reminder that I need to keep patient safety at the forefront of all my practice. In future, I'll work on my interpersonal skills to help build my confidence and be more assertive in my communication. I plan to attend the university workshops dealing with such issues. I think it would also be helpful to regularly reflect upon The Code (NMC 2015a) to ensure I meet the required standards. As I may frequently work as part of a team involving doctors, I believe it would be beneficial to familiarise myself with the General Medical Council Members' Code of Conduct (2013) in their Good Medical Practice documentation so that I've a better understanding of the role we all play as healthcare professionals.

3RS – RECAP, REVIEW, REFLECT

Do things seem clearer now? Good! Now log your learning. Don't make the mistake of thinking that once the placement is over then reflective practice is over. It isn't! That's just the start of your professional practitioner journey – you need to be constantly engaged in your thinking, feeling and logging. Remember, logging your thoughts isn't simply reflecting for reflective practice sake; it's a reflexive process of self-enquiry, a learning journey (Johns 2013) that should cement your learning and take account of your professional responsibilities and desires to become the practitioner you set out to be the first day you determinedly walked through those university doors. So, look at reflection as this unique learning opportunity and not as an overwhelming exercise that feels like a burden! That is, if you're aiming to become a positive professional practitioner who's not afraid to self-question and accept mentors' (or others') feedback to become more self-aware, and so adopt a different, more improved approach to your daily practice. Let's be honest then, when asking: What…

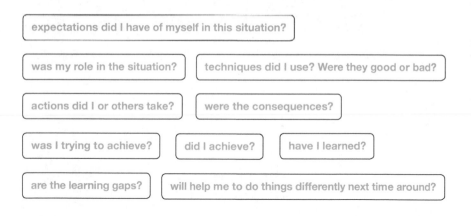

expectations did I have of myself in this situation?

was my role in the situation?   techniques did I use? Were they good or bad?

actions did I or others take?   were the consequences?

was I trying to achieve?   did I achieve?   have I learned?

are the learning gaps?   will help me to do things differently next time around?

If you enjoy it, note it; if you don't – note that too. Remember, to learn effectively and make the process useful, note the good, the bad and reasonably okay bits. Oh, and the why of all this.

Struggling with the idea of reflection? Not sure how to tackle it at first? Then get together with your peers, get support, give support, feed into the feedback and synthesise all this with your own thinking, feeling, learning. Don't forget – the more you share, the better you understand; and the more you reflect, the more critical your reflection. Reflective practice enriched!

ACTIVITY 7.3   LOOK BACKWARDS TO MOVE FORWARDS

As a group, exchange information, share opinions and views, and identify one key area each, where looking back can help you to move forwards in future practice and learning.

What you did, how you did it and why
What you've learned from your reflection
How you're feeling about what you've learned – positive, negative, concerned
What you're thinking about how you're feeling
What you've learned from this
What you feel is relevant to your practitioner learning process
What difficulties did you experience?
What internal or external factors contributed to this?
How did you solve these difficulties?
What impact did your action have on you, on others?
What theory applies to what happened?
Is there something you wished you'd known before starting the tasks?
What are the gaps in your learning?
How do you feel about the gaps?
What needs to improve to close the gaps?
Is there anything you'd do differently next time?

That done, now identify a few activities for your group to reflect upon over the next few weeks and share in your discussion room. Remember, be mindful of the NMC *Social Media Guidance* (2016)! When you come to reflect, see how much you've progressed in those few weeks. Now do you see the sense in what you're doing?

Remember, if you're good at reflecting on your current practice then you'll surely become a good lifelong professional practitioner! So don't make the mistake of completing your entire placement before reflecting on how it all went. Do that and your thoughts and feelings are lost to the wind. Take 10 minutes each day, log your feeling, thinking and learning reflections as you go along and see your learning landscape take shape. Sort out your ideas and thoughts and formulate new ones so that theory makes sense in practice and your practice makes sense in theory (Gribben 2012).

Want to improve future performance as a nurse or midwife? Then don't be afraid to revisit the 3Rs often, and be clear about how you'll use the new information, knowledge, skills, techniques in all future practice. Oh, and to nurture your learning potential and make connections between your experience and your existing knowledge, use your preferred learning style (Chapter 1) to positively reflect on your reflection. Isn't it interesting to take stock of your progress, to note how your skills have grown, and most of all how your perception and approach have changed from classroom theory to placement practice? See the gap closing between theory and practice? All make sense now?

THE REFLECTIVE PRACTITIONER – CONTINUING PROFESSIONAL DEVELOPMENT

We don't stop thinking about what we're doing or how we do things once we've graduated. Reflection doesn't suddenly stop once we've qualified, registered as a nurse or midwife, and landed that job! No, it continues long into our working days. It's the only way we can professionally develop and learn; and it's the only way we can positively contribute to change in the patient-care process. So by demonstrating your professional commitment you'll enhance your practice and create opportunities to influence change in the wider nursing or midwifery practice (www.flyingstart.scot.nhs.uk/learning-programmes/research-for-practice/research-and-evidence-based-practice-everyones-responsibility/).

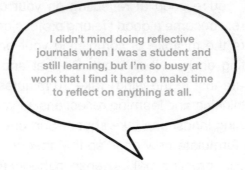

Sure you can – Pause! Breathe! Reflect! Take time! Place yourself in the present moment and adopt mindfulness in your reflection (Johns 2013). Watch the change!

Remember – as a qualified and registered practitioner with experience and a broad knowledge base, you're in a stronger position to make judgements on current practice, to make recommendations 'in relation to your professional responsibilities, ethical considerations and moral obligations' (Bulman and Schutz 2013: 87), and to make a difference to future patient care. Want to be that nurse or midwife who does make the difference? Then continually develop your reflective practice – learn to log and you'll log to learn, and let your reflective practice make a difference!

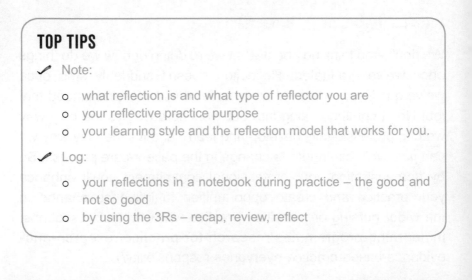

TOP TIPS

✔ Note:

- ○ what reflection is and what type of reflector you are
- ○ your reflective practice purpose
- ○ your learning style and the reflection model that works for you.

✔ Log:

- ○ your reflections in a notebook during practice – the good and not so good
- ○ by using the 3Rs – recap, review, reflect

- o your information-gathering process, e.g. books, articles, short courses attended
- o discussion (online or face-to-face), websites, media – at the end of each placement activity.

✓ Take 10 minutes each day to log your ELG.
✓ Reflect on your reflection on the same day and time each week.
✓ Colour code each information section and file your ELG.
✓ Develop a follow-up plan for your learning gaps.
✓ Build a raft using foam logs; pin on your reflection post-its to map your progress.
✓ Role play and share reflective experiences with your peers.
✓ Do some free writing to practise your reflection.
✓ Think out loud and record your reflection.
✓ Introduce graphics, pictures, symbols, colours, mind maps to your reflection.
✓ Write a task with supporting quotes or comments from literature on the left hand side of your journal and action or reflection on the right hand side.
✓ Write about the same event at in-action and on-action points and note the differences.
✓ Try out in-action and on-action reflection with different events.
✓ Practise mindfulness in reflection.

So those are the tips, but don't forget your toolkit at the end of the book!

FURTHER READING

Bassot, B. (2013) *The Reflective Journal*. Hampshire: Palgrave Macmillan.

Moon, J. (1999) *Reflection in Learning and Professional Development*. London: Kogan Page.

Skills You Need 'Reflective practice': www.skillsyouneed.com/ps/reflective-practice.html

Thompson, S. and Thompson, N. (2008) *The Critically Reflective Practitioner*. Hampshire: Palgrave Macmillan.

8 MAKING THEORY MAKE SENSE IN CLINICAL PRACTICE

⟹ Taught theory and practice realities – making it all make sense
⟹ Transferable skills – student to practitioner, clinic to clinic
⟹ 5Rs – recap, review, reflect, revisit, refresh

 CHAPTER OVERVIEW

Using the 5Rs process, this chapter helps you to consolidate your learning, bringing theory and practice together so it all makes sense. If you know how to bring together what you learn from the books and the lectures with what you practise on placement then you'll surely become a knowledgeable, safe and confident professional.

- Taught theory and practice realities – making it all make sense
- Transferable skills – student to practitioner, clinic to clinic
- 5Rs – recap, review, reflect, revisit, refresh

  - o Recap
  - o Review
  - o Reflect
  - o Revisit
  - o Refresh

- Top tips

TAUGHT THEORY AND PRACTICE REALITIES – MAKING IT ALL MAKE SENSE

Taught theory, practice realities – is there really such a difference? Well sometimes there can be, depending on the service demands, practices adopted in a specific area of nursing or midwifery within a specific organisation or region, and, of course, there's always the progressive nature of patient care, the expectations of patients, their carers and families, as well as your need to respond to meet the professional standards (NMC 2015a). Then there's the fact that some regional healthcare settings may be more advanced in their thinking and practice, have more available or disposable resources, and so be more able to carry out diverse institutionally tailored research projects that provide Evidence-based practice (EBP) recommendations; new ways of doing things supported by different systems and processes that can facilitate these new ideas. On top of that there's the reality of managing to respond to nursing and midwifery care delivery in remote and rural settings, where the very geographical nature of the landscape brings its own set of challenges, with patients often having to travel to receive care, healthcare practitioners often working in isolation, and the changing care needs of an often ageing, sometimes isolated population (NHS Scotland 2007). That's the reality! Let's start with you though.

You walked through the university doors highly motivated, your goal firmly in mind. We've taught you; you've learned. Then there's the fact that you come to your nursing and midwifery practice with sound knowledge, skills, values and beliefs – your point of reference in the application of theory to practice. Some of the theory you've learned will make perfect sense in practice, other aspects less so. Making it all make sense though is what counts. So how do you join the dots together to see the bigger picture in the tapestry of caring for your patients, while making sense of the 'why this' and 'not that' aspect of your practice? How do you weave your new knowledge and skills into practice while responding to the clinical setting demands? How does the way you're managed and mentored affect your approach to your patient care? Lots of questions, I know, but being aware of the diverse nature of your profession and the necessity of making the theory make sense in clinical practice (George 2010; Bryar and Sinclair 2011), and the consequences when it doesn't, should help you do a good job on the job.

As professionals, we do all we can do to improve the care and service we provide for our patients, often working alongside other healthcare professionals to adopt a holistic approach to our care delivery. Take, for example, the stroke patient who requires support from the doctor, nurse, radiographer, physiotherapist, speech and language therapist, occupational therapist, carer and social worker – so many professions providing crucial support at key stages in a patient's care. Working alongside other professionals during the course of your student journey should – if you grasp the learning opportunities – enrich your own professional practice. Think of the knowledge! Sound knowledge underpins safe practice, which in turn informs new knowledge (Hall 2005; WHO 2011). We know that; that's why we're reflective practitioners! So let your knowledge be as dynamic as the profession you've signed up to; learn from the past to improve the future; exercise professional accountability (NMC 2015a). Well that's the theory; what about the practice?

While theory gives you the foundation of nursing and midwifery practice, many of the practical things you carry out in service delivery can only be learned on placement, or when you start working as a fully registered nurse or midwife. So observe, ask, learn, practise. There's no other way to learn safe and efficient handover, for example, or to understand how theatre procedures differ from ward procedures, or even outpatient clinic procedures. It's only when you see things in reality and question that you really learn. Remember, there's power in questioning – stop questioning and you stop learning!

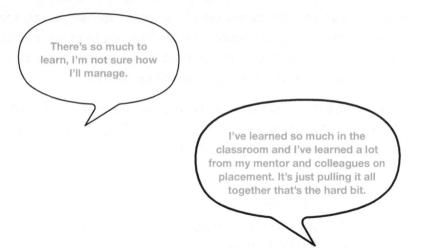

It will pull together, trust me! Somehow it will all make sense and you'll understand why you learned the things you did and why you do things the way you do. Look on your practice learning placement as the place to put your knowledge to the test, concerning the reality of patient care; where you've the opportunity to apply theoretical concepts to practical patient care; where you can observe, question, explore, and show your professionalism. It's where you're exposed to different cultures, patient demands and expectations; where you'll have to deal with emotionally charged or crisis situations, practise your communication skills, establish boundaries, and show you can remain calm under pressure (Stone 2011). It's where your beliefs, values and assumptions are put to the test; where you'll learn to identify ethical issues and understand how to deal with them. In your practice learning placement, you'll work as part of a team, learn to keep records and how to carry out effective handovers (Scovell 2010). You'll be mentored and supported, your commitment measured and your professional attitude and behaviour scrutinised, as determined by The Code (NMC 2015a).

Your practice learning placement is where you'll monitor your progress as a professional as you see the bigger picture of the theory–practice connection. The knowledge you've built up informs how you do things on placement, and what you learn there informs how you approach your learning in class and your future practice. So the learning continues, even long into your professional development days (see Chapter 12).

Your practice learning placement is also the place where we'll monitor you, recording your progress in your Ongoing Achievement Record (OAR) to ensure you achieve:

- your learning outcomes
- your fitness to practise, and
- the NMC competencies so you can register as a qualified nurse or midwife (NMC 2015a).

ACTIVITY 8.1   REFLECT ON YOUR KNOWLEDGE AND YOUR PRACTICE

What's the same; what's different? Note it! Consider how you'll bridge the theory–practice connection gap – note it!

So that's it then. You've come with your knowledge, values and beliefs. You monitor your progress; we monitor it too. Oh, but it doesn't stop there. What about the skills you bring – ever considered how they all fit in? Remember, skills are just as important as knowledge when it comes to practice, so let's take a look at their added value.

TRANSFERABLE SKILLS – STUDENT TO PRACTITIONER, CLINIC TO CLINIC

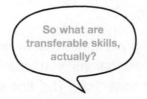

So what are transferable skills, actually?

I guess the best way to describe a transferable skill in nursing and midwifery is to say that it's a skill not restricted to one specific job, role or clinical situation (RNAO Careers in Nursing, http://careersinnursing.ca/new-grads-and-job-seekers/career-services/career-mapping). It's something you can carry from student days through to professional practice, and from one clinical situation to another – adaptable, versatile, useful skills that can help you settle into your new role and situation with relative ease, even if you're just at the start of your practice learning placements. Some are aptitudes – things you're naturally good at; others are acquired and developed through frequent practice. Then, as you grow in confidence and develop in your professional practice, the knowledge and experience you gain from the various clinical settings you've worked in, from the interactions you've had with other healthcare professionals and the continual professional development opportunities you undertake, should improve your skills even more. Added to that are the inherent qualities you bring to this caring profession, the qualities that make you 'you', the ones that led you to nursing or midwifery in the first place – compassion, care, empathy, integrity – those qualities that give added value to all you do in facilitating good patient care.

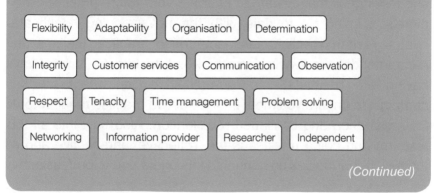

⚠ ACTIVITY 8.2   PORTABLE SKILLS – NAME YOURS

So whether aptitude or acquired skills, brainstorm with your peers to identify the transferable skills you'll carry with you from student learning to professional practice. Colour yours:

Flexibility	Adaptability	Organisation	Determination
Integrity	Customer services	Communication	Observation
Respect	Tenacity	Time management	Problem solving
Networking	Information provider	Researcher	Independent

(Continued)

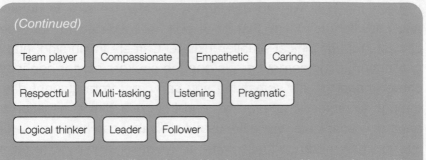

(Continued)

Team player   Compassionate   Empathetic   Caring

Respectful   Multi-tasking   Listening   Pragmatic

Logical thinker   Leader   Follower

Now profile your skills and consider how you could carry these with you from one clinical setting to another, from your student practice to qualified practitioner days. How transferable are these skills in different situations? Note it!

So you've considered your theoretical knowledge and its application to practice, you've looked at your transferable skills, now let's look at how you can bring it all together using the 5Rs. Oh, and remember to consider The Code (NMC 2015a) when working through these 5Rs. Do that and it should all surely make sense!

5RS – RECAP, REVIEW, REFLECT, REVISIT, REFRESH

Nursing and midwifery are demanding professions. Of course, you've understood that; it involves juggling family life, 'classroom' theory, practice learning placements, mentor meetings, personal study, assessments, reflecting on your practice and feedback, and feeding all that forward to improve your future practice. Then there's keeping up to date with the never-ending healthcare-related research with its evidence-based practice, findings and recommendations (www.nice.org.uk/). Add into the mix always having to be mindful of The Code (NMC 2015a), with its four key domains, to ensure you meet their fitness to practise requirements for registration and continued revalidation. Also built into all this learning and doing process is the 'reflective' perspective and all the new opportunities and benefits this offers you to professionally develop. Yes, it's demanding! But you can do it! The skills you learn as a student will give you a strong foundation as a professional practitioner. So keep your finger on the pulse, use the 5Rs as a self-assessment feedback tool to help you make sense of the theory–practice connection.

> But I'm so busy on placement, it takes me all my time completing my placement competency booklet. I'm not sure I'll manage anything extra!

Busy or not, you still need to find time to complete the booklet, do you not? It's crucial you do, so think – when better to take a little extra time to work through the 5Rs (see explanations below). So whether you complete this daily, weekly or at the end of each placement, embrace the learning opportunity and all it has to offer your professional development.

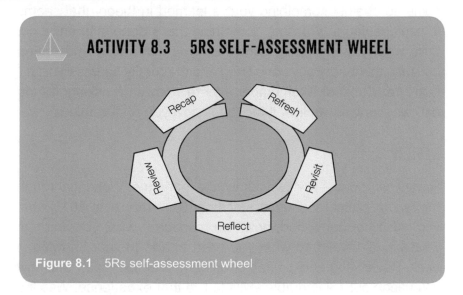

ACTIVITY 8.3   5RS SELF-ASSESSMENT WHEEL

Figure 8.1   5Rs self-assessment wheel

RECAP

You're about to go on placement. You'll be aware of the setting. So how do you plan to prepare? I guess a good place to start is to do some pre-placement preparation such as talking to others who've been on the same placement about the practicalities of getting there, the mentoring and the management set-up, plus the types of patients and care needed on placement so you can read up on care-related theory. Next, chat to your mentor about your placement so you can plan your placement commitments and duties, and have in place any support you'll need for your dyslexia or hearing impairment, for example. Then as you start working through your practice learning placements, recap on the specific practice-related theory and the knowledge you've acquired and see how it relates to what you're actually doing. So, if your place-ment is in neonatal care then it makes sense to recap on neonatal care-related theory. Can you see how all the knowledge you've acquired clicks into place when you're 'doing the learning' out in the community or on the ward? Can you see why you had to learn the subjects you did? You've recapped and achieved the theory–practice connection and it all makes sense! Then it happens – you come up against something you've learned in theory that seems to confuse you in practice. Something that's done differently, not quite what you expected, something you don't quite understand because the theory says one thing and the reality seems to differ? Don't fret! Just ask. Remember – there's power in asking; it's the only way forward really – it facilitates how you review things.

REVIEW

Review your day – review your lived experience. Working through the various clinical scenarios, storyboard (Lillyman et al. 2011) what you did, what happened, how you managed, what you learned, what you did well and what you need to add to your knowledge bank. Review the unexpected or different practice reality and how you used your transferable skills to live that experience. Was it a positive outcome? If so, what contributed to that? If not, is there anything you could have done differently? Reflect!

REFLECT

Reflecting should come easily to you – after all you're doing this all the time – but give it some real attention this time around; you're trying to make sense of everything in practice after all. This is your best chance to get it right. So read over old reflective journals, placement competency booklets and on-going achievement records, reflect on your previous reflections and feedback, identify what you need to polish up on, ask questions, make use of online resources, make use of your peers and team – find solutions. What have you learned from today's experience? What have been the joys and the challenges? Make every future day on placement a new and exciting learning experience not a mundane repeated one! Want to get it right? Then revisit your knowledge bank, revisit your clinical setting reality.

REVISIT

We can't know everything – that would be impossible, you're still learning after all – so expect some gaps. In fact, where there's evidence-based research, new findings and new ways of working to meet the ever-evolving service delivery, there will always be new things to learn – new knowledge, new skills (www.nice.org.uk/). This is what makes the nursing and midwifery profession exciting, interesting and exceedingly rewarding. You're at the cutting edge of the 'new' in healthcare. The key is to fill in those gaps by learning, embracing and adopting this 'new' so you make a difference to your own professional practice and to patient care. Not sure how best to approach that? Well, think of the theory–practice connection – in practice reality, what do you not know that you thought you did?

More than a few things? Then use the GapMap Bridge (Figure 8.2) to identify your gaps:

- Red (what you urgently need to work on to connect theory and practice).
- Amber (what's necessary to connect fairly soon so theory makes sense in clinical practice).
- Green (what's useful for you to work on so you understand the connection – but can wait for a few weeks).

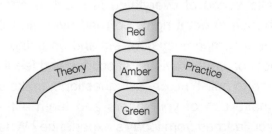

Figure 8.2 GapMap Bridge

Re-learn if you have to and plug the gaps, progressing from Green to Amber to Red. Facilitate professionally safe patient care – revisit, re-learn and you'll refresh service delivery.

REFRESH

What's all this about, I hear you say. Listen, refresh can be looked at in two ways:

- actively filling in the gaps so your knowledge joins up with the reality of practice, and by connecting this to new knowledge and skills
- taking a fresh look at the way you practise and breathing fresh new life into this by adjusting what you do and how.

Refresh all this and you'll refresh your own well-being (Hamilton et al. 2015). That's important too! Oh, and the well-being of those you care for. Even more important!

As a final reflective practice for yourself, look at each of the four domains of the 2015a NMC Code separately. Note the things you're good at and how you can build on these in practice. Note also the things you'd like to learn more about, something for your Continuing Professional Development (CPD) (see Chapter 12). Oh, and when doing all that note the things that clearly tie up with the legal and ethical aspects so that at the end of the day you can go home safe in the knowledge that you've been highly professional in delivering a sterling service to those under your care.

> ### ACTIVITY 8.4   ALWAYS LEARNING, ALWAYS CONNECTING
>
> Create a small network group where you can message each other securely, bearing in mind the NMC *Social Media Guidance* (2016) – identify theory–practice gaps, ask questions and provide solutions and overall support for each other. Refresh the way you learn – refresh the way you practise!

So you've made the most of your practice learning placements – the theory has finally met the practice; you're glad you took that first step through the university doors; you've made the most of the tools and support you've been given, you're glad you've stayed 'on course' and, of course, glad the hard work has finally paid off and you're about to graduate and register as a fully qualified nurse or midwife.

That's you, this is us.

Sure, we know it's a demanding profession – but from your first day to your final day, you've shown us both in class and on placement that you've the knowledge and skills necessary to become a confident, competent and compassionate nurse or midwife. You've met the NMC competencies (2009; 2010). So I guess with all that we can safely say, this is definitely the right profession for you!

TOP TIPS

✔ Practise the 5Rs daily, weekly, at the end of a clinical placement.
✔ Reflect on the NMC competencies when working through the 5Rs self-assessment wheel.
✔ Create a GapMap Bridge of what you need to learn using the Red, Amber, Green scaling system.
✔ If things don't seem to make sense on placement because they're different, ask your mentor to explain.
✔ Form a peer support network.
✔ Note the theory–practice differences in a pocket notebook.

So those are the tips, but don't forget your toolkit at the end of the book!

FURTHER READING

Colley, S. (2003) 'Nursing theory: its importance to practice', *Nursing Standard*, 17(46): 33–37.

Landa, J. and Lopez-Safra, E. (2010) 'The impact of emotional intelligence on nursing: an overview', *Psychology*, 1: 50–58.

McCormack, B. and McCance, T. (2010) *Person-Centred Theory and Practice*. West Sussex: Wiley-Blackwell.

NHS England (2016) *Care, Compassion, Competence, Communication, Courage, Commitment: Compassion in Practice – One Year On*. Leeds: NHS England/Nursing Directorate.

FITNESS TO PRACTISE – HOW TO BE A SAFE AND PROFESSIONAL NURSE OR MIDWIFE

⟹ Social media and your 'online self'
⟹ Duty of care, advocacy and whistleblowing
⟹ Safeguarding and protecting vulnerable groups
⟹ Patient safety and infection control
⟹ Achieving and maintaining your nursing and midwifery competencies

CHAPTER OVERVIEW

This chapter explores some of the key issues associated with being a safe and professional nurse or midwife. It doesn't matter which field of nursing practice you're studying (adult health, child health, learning disabilities or mental health), and it doesn't matter that midwifery is considered as a separate field of practice with its independent professional requirements – there are a number of core values, attitudes and ethical issues which all nurses and midwives need to be aware of. Focusing on 'fitness to practise', this chapter emphasises the importance of upholding the principles of the NMC Code (2015a)

(Continued)

(Continued)

and understanding the importance of achieving outcomes and competencies, to become a safe and professional clinical practitioner. To help you through this maze of requirements, we've broken the chapter down into 'bite-size' chunks, focusing on specific topics.

- Social media and your 'online self'
- Duty of care, advocacy and whistleblowing

  o Duty of care
  o Advocacy
  o Whistleblowing

- Safeguarding and protecting vulnerable groups
- Patient safety and infection control

  o Patient safety
  o Infection control

- Achieving and maintaining your nursing and midwifery competencies
- Top tips

SOCIAL MEDIA AND YOUR 'ONLINE SELF'

Love it or loathe it, social media is a huge part of people's lives; we know that. It's here to stay! Used in the right way, it can be an effective communication tool. But a word of advice – in nursing and midwifery, you're following a professional code of practice so you'll need to use social media with caution (NMC 2016). So, we hear you asking, 'What do you mean? I can't use Facebook or Twitter or Snapchat?' Not at all! You can use these media – in fact, some universities will actively encourage you to set up a student group Facebook account where you can help each other with questions about the course and set up support networks. However, you must remember that now you're training to become a nurse or midwife you've a duty to protect the people you care for. The Code (NMC 2015a) states that nurses and midwives should: 'Use all forms of spoken, written and digital communication (including social media and networking sites) responsibly' (*The Code*, paragraph 20.10). The message seems clear enough, but you might well ask – what does 'using communication methods responsibly' mean? Good question! In essence, it means two things:

- You must follow the NMC guidance on using social media; and,
- You need to clearly understand the role and responsibilities you're taking on as a student nurse or midwife, in relation to caring for patients and their families.

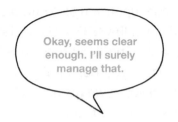

Okay, seems clear enough. I'll surely manage that.

Sure you will! But what it means in reality is you'll need to think about how, why, when and with whom you communicate, both personally and professionally. You'll have to think carefully about how personal discussions or activities might compromise the professional values we've already mentioned in Chapter 1, and which we'll discuss more fully in Chapter 10, as well as considering the consequences of such discussions or activities. As a student nurse or midwife, you've taken on a duty to protect your patients in all circumstances and situations. This means:

- not putting them in harm's way; and,
- making sure you maintain confidentiality at all times (NMC 2015a).

So, in your busy networking world of social media, it means never making reference to your work, your patients or to any patient-related activity in your postings. Think, they may be your online postings but you can never be sure who'll be reading what you write or post.

It wouldn't be the first time that a nurse or midwife has unwittingly made reference to a work situation which has resulted in a patient being identified! Remember – no naming and you'll have no shaming!

DUTY OF CARE, ADVOCACY AND WHISTLEBLOWING

DUTY OF CARE

When we talk about a duty of care, we're really talking about legal responsibilities from both a personal and collective (your colleagues' and employers') viewpoint. The law of the country you're working in will impose a duty of care upon you as a nurse or midwife, indeed on any practitioner working in the NHS or in social care (RCN 2015b). This duty of care is a binding legal duty, which in practice means you're obligated to ensure you don't put your patients at unnecessary risk, either through your own actions or by delegating duties to other team members. You need to make sure everyone has both the knowledge and capability to undertake and perform the activity effectively. Remember, your duty of care is linked closely to the principles of ethical and professional practice (Chapter 10).

So, now you can see and understand that you've a responsibility to protect patients and deliver a high standard of care, while also being accountable to the NMC, your employer and yourself (Brooker and Waugh 2013). Does this feel somewhat overwhelming? Simply put the patient at the centre of your work, focus care around their best interests, and think about the potential consequences of your actions in daily practice, and you'll find it's all achievable.

ACTIVITY 9.1   THINKING ABOUT YOUR 'DUTY OF CARE'

Tell me – what are the key areas of responsibility for nurses and midwives as set out in the NMC Code (2015a)? Note this in your reflective diary for future reference.

One of the main ways to protect patients is by maintaining confidentiality, which is a crucially important part of nursing and midwifery practice. By following a code of confidentiality in nursing and midwifery practice, it's generally expected that all patient-related data is shared with fellow practitioners on a 'need-to-know' basis only (NMC 2015a). So be mindful of when, where and with whom you share any patient-related information. Be aware of your responsibilities to gain your patient's consent (this can be implicit when you're sharing information with the care team, or explicit where the patient gives verbal or written consent). Oh, and be aware of your need to understand the close relationship between respecting your patient's right to privacy and deciding what information can safely be shared or disclosed.

⚓ ACTIVITY 9.2   MAINTAINING CONFIDENTIALITY AND GAINING CONSENT

CASE SCENARIO

Robert is 67 years old and lives in a care home. He's a sociable man who gets on well with the majority of residents and staff. Recently, he's been attending hospital for investigations to discover the cause of a troublesome cough and lack of appetite. One of Robert's close friends in the care home is 62-year-old Mary who's concerned about him. She asks the Care Assistant what's wrong with Robert and what the doctor at the hospital had said. Mary says she wants to help him as his friend. As the Care Assistant has worked in the care home for a long time and so knows them both well, she tells Mary what was discussed at the hospital.

ACTIVITY

Use the above scenario to consider the NMC guidance on maintaining confidentiality and gaining consent. Identify whether it was acceptable for the Care Assistant to mention Robert's results to his close friend Mary.

ADVOCACY

When you undertake your 'duty of care' you're also working as an advocate for the patient. Advocating means you support your patients by making sure their rights are upheld, their voices are heard and their views are taken into consideration to help achieve the best outcome for them, without judging or giving your personal opinion (seAp 2015). It's about making sure that nursing and midwifery practice places the dignity, care and rights of each individual patient at its centre (NMC 2015a). Although it's essential for effective patient care, being an advocate isn't easy! In managing risk to ensure patient safety, you might just find yourself facing difficult or challenging situations in practice, which as 'the voice of the patient' you'll have to deal with and even report. It's not easy, we know, but when a patient's health and well-being isn't as good as it could be, they'll need someone else to speak up for them, advocate on their behalf – and that could mean you as the student nurse or midwife. The NMC (2015b) clearly states your responsibility to raise and act upon anything that causes you concern in relation to patient care. In rare situations, this might also mean that you'll need to breach confidentiality, in the best interest of the patient! So let's reflect on that one.

ACTIVITY 9.3   DISCLOSURE SITUATIONS

Referring back to the NMC Code (2015a) regarding confidentiality, can you identify the type of situations that might arise where nurses and midwives are allowed, or expected, to disclose patient information, and why? Note it!

WHISTLEBLOWING

In nursing and midwifery practice, there will be times when we're worried about a patient's care delivery or a colleague's poor practice at work. When this starts to raise questions about the principles and values of nursing and midwifery then we call this 'raising concerns' or 'whistleblowing' – the NMC's language for dealing with difficult situations (NMC 2015b). Let's face it, nobody really wants to be involved in reporting people, but when you're in the responsible (and privileged) position of caring for patients, you're obliged to make sure their well-being, safety and dignity is your first concern – even as a student. So familiarise yourself with the NMC 'whistleblowing' language and processes at the start of your career. Now, let's look at the sort of things that could cause concern and what you should do about them.

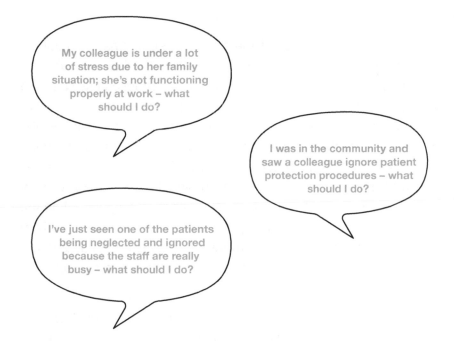

My colleague is under a lot of stress due to her family situation; she's not functioning properly at work – what should I do?

I was in the community and saw a colleague ignore patient protection procedures – what should I do?

I've just seen one of the patients being neglected and ignored because the staff are really busy – what should I do?

Well, you're working under a code of professional practice – correct? Then in all of these situations, you've a duty to report them. Fail to report and you'll be failing in your duty as a student nurse or midwife. You also have a 'duty of candour' (GMC/NMC 2015), which means that even if you only have a suspicion of poor care delivery, you're obliged to report it. That might simply involve reporting it to your mentor or to the nurse or midwife in charge, and asking them to deal with it. On very rare occasions, it might be serious enough for you to report it to the NMC! As the profession's governing body, the NMC want staff to feel protected and able to raise concerns without fear, so that patient care can be delivered safely and effectively. Their specific guidance covers both students and registered nurses and midwives alike; check out *Raising Concerns* (NMC 2015b: www.nmc.org.uk/standards/guidance/raising-concerns-guidance-for-nurses-and-midwives/) for more information.

SAFEGUARDING AND PROTECTING VULNERABLE GROUPS

Okay, we've just discussed the need to report unsafe situations and protect patients, all of which links into the issue of what we call 'safeguarding' in nursing and midwifery practice (RCN 2014a; 2015c). By now, you should be able to see that patient protection is a key focus of nursing and midwifery practice. Your responsibility is to ensure that people in your care are safe and aren't being subjected to any form of abuse or harm. So to make patient safety and well-being your primary concern, you'll work closely with colleagues from other disciplines such as social work, education and the third sector (our voluntary services and charitable bodies). Part of your responsibility also means that you need to understand safeguarding procedures so you can recognise and manage individual situations as they arise.

Within the UK, each of the four countries (England, Scotland, Wales and Northern Ireland) have slightly different procedures relating to patient protection in two areas:

- Protection and support of adults procedures; and,
- Separate procedures for the protection of children and young people.

The wide range of policies and legislation (Acts of Parliament) (Appendix 1) detail the legislative policies which nurses and midwives need to adhere to, according to the law of the land they're working in (Thurston 2013). As a guide, policies refer to the creation of guidance and best practice at local and national level, whereas legislation refers to the creation of laws which are made in statute to regulate activities and outline responsibilities at a national level. Sounds complicated? Then identify the safeguarding policy and legislation of the country you're working in and, to safeguard yourself as a professional, familiarise yourself with this so you understand your role and accountability for patient safety and well-being. Want to learn more than just 'familiarise' – then check out, 'Introduction to safeguarding for adults' (www. nmc.org.uk/standards/safeguarding/introduction-to-safeguarding-for-adults/).

PATIENT SAFETY AND INFECTION CONTROL

PATIENT SAFETY

So what do we mean by patient safety? Just keeping them from harm and looking after them? Not really, it's a bit more complicated than that. In fact, it's a whole subject of study in itself; something that you'll cover extensively in your undergraduate programme. As a start, let's note the variety of important factors that fall under the issue of 'patient safety'.

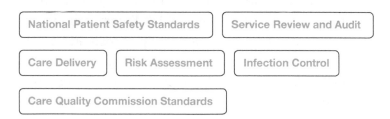

The National Patient Safety Agency (NPSA) plays an important role across the UK by trying to reduce the potential for exposing patients and families to unnecessary risk (NPSA 2004) by collecting information about any adverse or dangerous situations that happen in the healthcare setting – for example, medication errors, moving and handling issues or poor infection control techniques. These types of events are categorised into mild, moderate or severe risks, reported to the NPSA and then dealt with according to local policy. Even as a student nurse or midwife, you might witness unsafe situations. It's vital, therefore, that you understand the risk management reporting process within your placement area.

⚓ **ACTIVITY 9.4   RISK ASSESSMENT**

Make a mental note to yourself to ask what the risk management reporting process is in each practice learning placement you go to.

> But how will I learn about all this and know what to do?

Don't worry! This is something you'll explore in more detail as part of your study programme. We're not going to give you the information and just let you get on with it. No! We'll help you identify common tools that should help you confidently assess and evaluate clinical practice risks. During practice learning you might also be involved in the completion of risk assessments at some point in your programme, whether it's in the community setting with a patient requiring some assistive equipment or in the hospital where they're recovering from surgery and preparing to go home. It doesn't matter what the situation is or whether the risks are actual or just potential; the principles of assessment are the same and should follow the National Patient Safety Agency's *Seven*

Steps to Patient Care (NPSA 2004), to help reduce and manage all risks in the clinical setting.

Another important area of patient safety is making sure services are delivered effectively to meet patients' needs. The most efficient way to do this is through service reviews and audits that provide information to improve patient care and service delivery (Thurston 2013). As a student nurse or midwife, you might find yourself in the fortunate position of working alongside a mentor who's undertaking an audit of their service – to review and evaluate current practices and determine what does or doesn't work well. This will be an important and interesting learning opportunity for you, so make sure you grasp it!

Well, are you now starting to see how important it is to protect patients and keep them safe? How this ultimately contributes to their well-being? How everyone has a role to play, and how important your role is as a student nurse or midwife? Remember, this isn't only important for the patients themselves, it's also important from a professional and organisational perspective. Understand this when you're a student and you've understood it for life. Oh, and it's also helpful to be aware of who's responsible for monitoring standards of care delivery for patients, even as a student. So within the UK, patient safety regulations are a little different in each of the four countries. In England, the Care Quality Commission (CQC) plays a key role in reviewing and regulating the performance of all services and organisations in both social care and the NHS (CQC 2016). It not only sets standards which it expects to be met on a regular basis, it also provides reports about activity (good and bad) for governments and the public to review. In Wales, this role is played by the Care and Social Services Inspectorate (CSSIW 2016), and, in Northern Ireland, by the Regulation and Quality Improvement Authority (RQIA 2016). In Scotland, Healthcare Improvement Scotland (HIS 2016) takes responsibility for the quality and monitoring of NHS provision, while the Care Inspectorate (Care Inspectorate 2016) regulates social care and social work services.

INFECTION CONTROL

So what about infection control as part of patient safety? You're probably saying 'Oh yes, that's all to do with this MRSA stuff in the news…', and to a certain extent you'd be right, but there's much more to it than that! We've known about the importance of preventing the spread of infection since the days of Florence Nightingale in the 1800s, when she identified it as being the most important thing in helping soldiers recover from injuries in the Crimean War (George 2010). We've come a long way in our understanding about infection control since the 1800s. As student nurses or midwives, you'll spend a fair bit of your time (particularly in the first year) studying this topic to acquire a basic understanding of infection control, which you can then develop throughout your career. The main focus of this input is to understand how infection develops and how to prevent it spreading between patients and staff (RCN 2014b). You'll have heard of a 'chain reaction'. Well, in healthcare this is what we call the 'chain of infection' (Brooker and Waugh 2013).

When we talk about controlling the spread of infection, we refer to something called 'standard precautions' (WHO 2006); all nurses, midwives and fellow practitioners are expected to stringently follow these – for example, correct handwashing procedures, appropriate use of gloves and aprons, and protection against blood and body fluids. As a student nurse or midwife, you'll be working across a range of placement learning environments in the community setting and the acute hospital. You'll be working in care homes, day centres, nurseries, family centres, rehabilitation centres, medical/surgical wards, health centres – to name but a few. But wherever you're working, the standard principles of infection control still apply. Oh, and be aware – you'll be assessed on your ability to implement and follow the infection control guidelines. Want to check out some of the standards?

⚠ ACTIVITY 9.5   INFECTION CONTROL IN PRACTICE

Access the World Health Organisation (WHO) Infection Control Standard Precautions and 'Key Elements at a Glance' leaflet (WHO 2006) and note down the key elements for your practice (www.who.int/csr/resources/publications/4EPR_AM2.pdf).

Interesting, but want to read more? Then check out some evidence-based resources about infection control and prevention by the National Institute for Health and Care Excellence (NICE) and the Scottish Intercollegiate Guidelines Network (SIGN). Also check out the NHS Education for Scotland (NES) Breaking the Chain of Infection (2012a) interactive resource (www.nes.scot.nhs.uk/) and add it to your resource bank.

Okay, by now you're probably thinking – this is a bit too complicated; how am I going to understand all of this important information? As a student, it's crucially important to learn to understand the importance of infection control standards so you'll automatically begin to adopt the key principles of infection control in your everyday practice. It's a complex area, we know, but to help you understand it further, each of the four countries in the UK have their own Strategic Infection Control programmes, which relate to local and national policies (Department of Health 2008, revised 2015; Department of Health, Social Services and Public Safety 2011; Health Protection Scotland 2015; Public Health Wales 2014). While different terms and abbreviations are used in practice, the most common description you'll hear relates to Healthcare Associated Infections, also known as HCAIs or HAIs. As a student nurse or midwife, you'll be introduced to the HCAI or HAI 'toolkit' booklet, which you're expected to work through during your study programme. Do this and you'll surely develop knowledge and gain competencies in infection control management – essential components in becoming a registered nurse or midwife.

ACHIEVING AND MAINTAINING YOUR NURSING AND MIDWIFERY COMPETENCIES

Let's think back to Chapter 1 where we talked about the NMC, what it does and what it means to be a registered nurse or midwife. Do you remember the four requirements all student nurses or midwives need to achieve before they register?

- To be confirmed of good character and good health, meaning you're capable of safe practice without supervision.
- To have undertaken a specific number of theory hours.
- To have undertaken a specific number of practice hours.
- To have achieved clinical competencies, as assessed by your mentor.

Okay then, the achievement of clinical competencies is key to becoming registered as a nurse or midwife; it demonstrates your ability to link theory with practice as you provide evidence to support your clinical judgements and care delivery – in effect, it proves you *are* competent!

So let's just recap on what we mean by 'competence'. The NMC (2014) describes competence as having the skills and ability to practise safely and effectively without supervision. The RCN (2009) has produced a comprehensive resource relating to achieving competence within the NHS Knowledge Skills Framework (KSF) to help nurses and midwives develop understanding and demonstrate knowledge and skills.

Clear enough? But competencies don't just relate to students, not at all – they relate to every registered nurse and midwife throughout their working lives. To achieve the status of a registered professional nurse or midwife you must undertake, and successfully complete, a course of study that's been validated (approved) by the professional governing body – in this case the NMC. Once you've qualified as a nurse or midwife, you register your name with the NMC, pay a registration fee and from then on, you never stop learning! Not only are there new aspects of your job role to learn about, there are also standardised competencies and compulsory studies which you *have* to achieve every year – those little things we call mandatory updates. You never stop learning!

If you think back to the NMC Code (2015a), there are four key aspects of practice: prioritising people, practising effectively, preserving safety and promoting professionalism and trust. As a future nurse or midwife, you must have your name and qualifications recorded on the professional register to ensure you work within the Code, and have your practice monitored by a process called 'revalidation'. This means renewing your name on the register every three years by paying a specific revalidation fee (set by the NMC), and proving you take the profession seriously by reflecting on the role you're undertaking to deliver safe and effective practice. Understand the NMC requirements and you'll meet the revalidation criteria below:

- Complete 450 practice hours over a three-year period or 900 if revalidating as both a nurse and midwife.
- Complete 35 hours of Continuous Professional Development (CPD), including 20 hours participatory learning which must be clearly linked to the Code and its domains.
- Produce five pieces of practice-related feedback which reflect the domains of The Code.
- Produce five written reflective accounts relating to CPD and which also reflect the domains of practice.
- Produce a reflective discussion.
- Complete a good health and character declaration.
- Provide evidence of professional indemnity arrangements.
- Provide confirmation of all of the above through a signed declaration form from your chosen Confirmer, who must be a registered nurse or midwife.

(Adapted from NMC revalidation online)

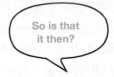

So is that it then?

Well no! As well as renewing your registration with the NMC every three years, you'll also have local competencies and updates to achieve within your employing organisation. These are usually repeated and achieved every year or two years, and will differ depending on where you work. Some updates are mandatory for all staff, such as efficient moving and handling, safe administration of medicines or resuscitation. Sometimes you'll complete additional or advanced competencies such as blood transfusion, administration of intravenous medication, or administration of cytotoxic medication. Again, depending on the role you're undertaking, they'll differ; for example, if you're a specialist nurse or an advanced nurse practitioner (ANP). Regardless of the role, you'll need to become familiar with the key competency requirements to ensure you provide care that's effective, safe and based on the best available evidence.

So a quick recap! There are many aspects to becoming a safe and professional nurse or midwife and, at this point in your career, all this will seem a bit complicated and quite daunting. Don't fret though. Simply remember – your ultimate aim is to provide evidence-based care which is patient-focused, safe and effective. Do this, and everything will fall into place as part of your daily routine in practice. Do this, and you're sure to adhere to the professional Code (NMC 2015a) and fulfil the professional requirements, whichever post and setting you find yourself working in.

TOP TIPS

✔ Highlight the key competencies – colour code.
✔ Mind map the NMC domains of practice – colour code.
✔ Brainstorm the pitfalls of poor infection control with your peers and discuss ways to improve your own practice.

> ✔ Note difficult situations in your pocket notebook and discuss with your mentor or manager.
> ✔ Role play a difficult situation with your peers and identify ways to handle issues professionally.
> ✔ Reflect on what you personally can learn from these situations and record this in your journal.

So those are the tips, but don't forget your toolkit at the end of the book!

FURTHER READING

Barksby, J. (2014) 'Service users' perceptions of student nurses', *Nursing Times*, 111(19): 23–25.

Galanti, G.A. (2008) *Caring for Patients from Different Cultures*, 4th edition. Pennsylvania: Pennsylvania University Press.

Kline, R. with Khan, S. (2013) *The Duty of Care of Healthcare Professionals.* Public World (www.publicworld.org/files/Duty_of_Care_handbook_April_2013.pdf).

NHS Education for Scotland (2012b) *Advanced Nursing Practice Toolkit: Legal and Ethics Guidance* (www.advancedpractice.scot.nhs.uk/legal-and-ethics-guidance.aspx).

10

EXPECTATIONS AND RESPONSIBILITIES IN NURSING AND MIDWIFERY CLINICAL PRACTICE

⟹ Expectations and responsibilities in nursing and midwifery practice
⟹ Performance – behaviour, values, moral beliefs and attitudes
⟹ The importance of ethics in nursing and midwifery practice
⟹ Leadership skills

 CHAPTER OVERVIEW

This chapter addresses some of the key expectations and responsibilities you're expected to meet as a nurse or midwife. Focusing on some of the key areas you'll need to develop skills in, it looks at performance and how behaviour, values, moral beliefs and attitudes can affect your clinical practice. It considers the importance of ethics in guiding you through your professional life, and the importance of 'getting it right' to ensure your care and clinical judgements are completely up to date and built upon the most recent evidence. The leadership skills of accountability, honesty and integrity are also addressed, as are the specific differences in supervision between nursing and midwifery practice.

- Expectations and responsibilities in nursing and midwifery practice
- Performance – behaviour, values, moral beliefs and attitudes
- The importance of ethics in nursing and midwifery practice
- Leadership skills

  o Key responsibilities

- Top tips

EXPECTATIONS AND RESPONSIBILITIES IN NURSING AND MIDWIFERY PRACTICE

So you're thinking this is all getting a little bit serious now aren't you? Expectations, responsibilities, leadership, ethics, integrity – oh no, how will I cope with it all? Is this really for me? Can I do all this? Sure you can! Trust me, once you're working in clinical practice, gaining and assimilating all that vast array of knowledge and putting it into action with your patients, you'll soon find it all 'magically' falls into place without thinking too much about it.

You automatically want to protect your patients, don't you? To care for them, make sure they come to no harm and basically do your best for them? And to do all this while upholding the principles of ethical and professional practice? Sure you do! Hold this view and you possess the very things that form the principles of ethical and professional practice; the very things that enable you to perform with integrity and develop solid leadership skills. Sure, there are some specific terms you'll need to know and some background you'll need to understand, but essentially ethical and professional practice all comes down to being respectful and mindful of people's opinions, their backgrounds, socialisation and their personal beliefs. It's about putting the patient at the centre of everything you do and following the professional Code (NMC 2015a) you signed up to. So let's look at this in a little more detail...

PERFORMANCE – BEHAVIOUR, VALUES, MORAL BELIEFS AND ATTITUDES

Oh, so you want to be a nurse or a midwife then? It's not an easy profession, you know that – but you also know it's an extremely rewarding one; an exciting profession with so many different career options open to you. And to be a successful nurse or midwife, you'll need to make efficient and effective decisions about patient care – but how do you know they're right?

Well, apart from making sure you're using the best available evidence, as discussed in Chapter 5, you'll need to rely quite heavily on your personal values and beliefs to make sound moral judgements or decisions about the many issues you face in practice. Values? Yes values! The very things we turn to when making a decision, a judgement or even when facing a dilemma – moral or otherwise. They're important to us as individuals, we pick them up during our lifetime; they become part of who we are (Egan 2013). Essentially they're the ideals, customs or beliefs that form part of the 'totally unique you'; the things that drive your behaviour, attitudes and thought processes. Want to look at this a little closer? Then complete the following, jotting down your answers in your reflective diary.

ACTIVITY 10.1   THE 'TOTALLY UNIQUE YOU'

List your own personal values and beliefs about life and life issues using the headings below.

Your value/belief	Where did it come from?	Has it changed over time and why?
[Example] Respect	Family upbringing	No, I still think it's important

Influenced by our upbringing, education, socialisation, religious or political beliefs, in short our general life experience, we recognise values as something good or worthwhile. Oh, and depending on the situations we're exposed to, we'll find that some of these values may be fixed, or some may change over time. We'll not see the change but we'll be conscious of it, particularly when one or other situation challenges them in our professional practice as a nurse or midwife. Think about the issue of conscientious objection, where a nurse or midwife objects to caring for a patient who's undergoing a termination of pregnancy. For some people, being part of this activity conflicts with a strong personal value or their moral/religious beliefs which they can't compromise on. This is covered under The Code (NMC 2015a) and allows nurses or midwives to lodge their conscientious objection with a senior member of staff, and to avoid participating without recrimination. So that's an example of a fixed value, but what about flexible ones; you know, those values which may change over time? Maybe it's your values about health and well-being, about not being overweight and eating healthily. Think about how you value your health in general. You feel it's important; you value your health? Of course you do! You try to eat well, do enough exercise, avoid too much of the unhealthy things (sugar, smoking, alcohol) – and yet sometimes you 'fall off' the healthy lifestyle, depending on the situation you're in. This doesn't mean you don't value your health does it? Of course not! It just means you make a personal choice based upon the information you have or the situation you're in. This relates to patients too!

Think about people who struggle with maintaining a healthy lifestyle due to their personal situation or condition – the fact that they don't meet strict criteria and follow best practice guidelines all the time doesn't mean they don't value their health does it? As a nurse or midwife, your values about health and well-being may change over time, as you begin to understand some of the more complex influences patients face in relation to maintaining general health. This is where being non-judgemental is important – remember The Code (NMC 2015a) states that nurses and midwives should work in an equitable and non-judgemental way. That's where being aware of, and understanding, people's individual personal values becomes important because as human beings we'll all judge things according to our own views. However, it's what we do with them and how we work with them to make sure they don't interfere with patient care that's important. Remember this and you'll capture the crucially important factor in being a successful nursing or midwifery practitioner. See the connection? When we're challenged, we return 'home' to the 'totally unique you'! Okay those are the values, now what about the moral beliefs?

Well, this is another important aspect of nursing and midwifery practice as you'll be challenged in lots of different situations, many of which will be new to you, and you'll turn to your values and moral viewpoint to make sense of things and make decisions. Morals are to do with honesty, making choices, being fair and valuing people. Beliefs are the things that make sense of our world and are important in shaping our behaviour as they come from what people tell us to be true, often when we're young. We either accept or question the information we're given, but, nevertheless, this information can shape our behaviour and influence our values. Think about freedom of choice, of access to basic healthcare – depending on your culture, where you live and how you've been brought up, your values and moral beliefs about these issues will differ, sometimes quite dramatically. So you can see that values and moral beliefs are closely linked to each other and have originated from different sources/people over time.

Okay, feel you've got the message then? Of course, you'll learn more about all this during your study programme, and as you professionally develop, you'll learn to link professional expectations and responsibilities with personal values and beliefs. Do that and you'll enhance your ability to deliver compassionate and sensitive patient care. Excellent – no worries then! Well, not quite – fail to do that and you'll restrict that delivery; the very one you signed up to provide! So let's check your understanding of all this by reflecting on the following. Jot down your thoughts and responses in your reflective diary.

⚠ **ACTIVITY 10.2   CASE SCENARIO**

A 2-year-old child is admitted to the ward you're working in. She's a bit unkempt, not thriving very well and has a high temperature. The little girl is quite distressed, often crying for her mum – a young, single parent who hasn't visited very often since her daughter's admission.

Now tell me your thoughts. What's your reaction to her mum when she does arrive? How do you deal with all this?

In this case, it would be easy to judge wouldn't it, because your own attitude and opinions come into play? You might find it quite shocking that the mother isn't there, you might have discussions with staff about the lack of parent contact, and you might well make your own decisions about the little girl's mother based on this situation. At this point, if you allow your personal opinion (based upon your personal values) to go unchecked, you run the risk of affecting your professional relationship with the mother and ultimately the little girl.

Let's reflect on the situation again. Is there anything you could do differently to deal with this? Any information you'd want to find out before making a judgement or offering your opinion? Reflect and note! Of course, there's another way of thinking about all this; one that compromises neither your personal nor your professional values. As a start, you could acknowledge your thoughts and feelings and then take a step into 'reflective action' mode (see Chapter 7). Ask yourself:

Okay – why isn't the mother visiting?

Any specific reason?

Why is the little girl unkempt and not thriving?

Is her mother unwell?

Are there other pressures/children at home?

What sort of support does this young, single mother have?

What are her previous hospital experiences?

Reflecting in this way, you're putting the patient at the centre and considering all the other factors that contribute to them being in hospital or requiring care. Of course, while this is an example of a child as a patient, you can apply the same key principles to a patient of any age – a pregnant woman, newborn baby, teenager, a middle-aged or older person. It really doesn't matter about the age, it's about putting the patient at the centre of your care and doing your professional best for them.

By considering such situations, you can hopefully begin to see how your attitudes and beliefs are shaped by your underlying values. It's really important to understand this, as it forms the basis of who you are and how you both accept and react to people and situations. As nurses and midwives, you'll be coming into contact with a lot of people from many different backgrounds (cultural, ethnic, socio-economic), so it's crucially important to treat everyone the same, regardless of your own views (Landa and Lopez-Safra 2010). It's a tall order, we know, especially as we all like to think that our own views are the right ones. Be aware though – as a nurse or a midwife undertaking patient care, you're required to put these to one side. Your patient is key!

As a profession, nursing and midwifery has its own set of values (NMC 2015a), showing it has a collective responsibility to guide nurses and midwives in both maintaining patient safety and promoting health and well-being. This is what we would call a deontological approach to healthcare delivery – meaning that there are some rules which are totally inflexible and so must be adhered to regardless of your own values and beliefs. So, for example, a patient you're working with discloses information which indicates they may be a danger to themselves. You're mindful of the need to maintain confidentiality (NMC 2015a), while at the same time being mindful of the need to adhere to section 5.4 of the Code: 'you must share necessary information with other healthcare professionals and agencies, only when the interests of patient safety and public protection override the need for confidentiality'. In this case, you'd have no choice but to report the information to a senior colleague – just one example of an 'inflexible' rule, as set down by the NMC.

By following The Code, you'll develop a sense of professional identity to guide you in learning what to do and how to do it, what to believe and what to value.

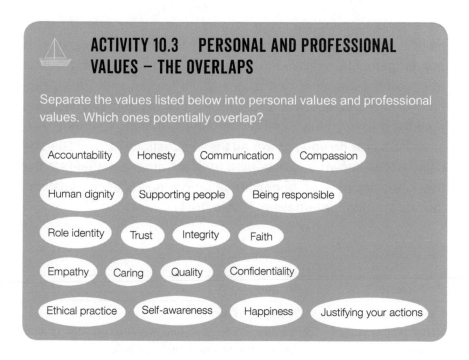

ACTIVITY 10.3   PERSONAL AND PROFESSIONAL VALUES – THE OVERLAPS

Separate the values listed below into personal values and professional values. Which ones potentially overlap?

Accountability   Honesty   Communication   Compassion

Human dignity   Supporting people   Being responsible

Role identity   Trust   Integrity   Faith

Empathy   Caring   Quality   Confidentiality

Ethical practice   Self-awareness   Happiness   Justifying your actions

See the value in your values, even the overlaps? So how do they translate when dealing with ethics in reality?

THE IMPORTANCE OF ETHICS IN NURSING AND MIDWIFERY PRACTICE

You'll notice we've listed 'ethical practice' as a value – something else you'll need to be aware of. Why? Well, like moral beliefs, 'ethics' are closely linked to 'values' and are concerned with the way nurses and midwives manage and conduct themselves, both personally and professionally. Practising ethically means practising within the law of the country you're working in and following the professional code. Don't worry, you'll learn much more about this during your study programme, but for now we'll introduce you to the basic essentials to help you understand their link with nursing and midwifery practice.

As a guiding principle, your job as a nurse or midwife is to deliver and facilitate equitable and compassionate care in a non-judgemental way. Sounds easy doesn't it? But what about the potentially complicated issues you'll face in your daily practice? You might well ask yourself: What's my role? What's the right thing to do? How can I be certain I'm making the right decisions? So how do you answer all these questions? Easy! Start by using a well-known and accepted ethical framework that lists the five key principles of 'beneficence', 'non-maleficence', 'justice', 'autonomy' and 'paternalism' (Table 10.1).

Table 10.1 Ethical framework principles

Principle	Meaning
Beneficence	A duty to do good
Non-maleficence	A duty to do no harm and to safeguard your patients
Justice	Consider everyone's interests fairly
Autonomy	Ability to make decisions yourself without the help of others
Paternalism	When you need to overrule someone's actions or wishes to prevent harm coming to them

Take note: 'paternalism' is only ever justified if the potential for harm to a patient outweighs the need to lose their independent decision-making ability. Take note, too: all this is just a 'framework' to help staff make decisions based on the well-being of patients; it's not a prescriptive decision-making formula to give you the answers. Nevertheless, we hope it helps. Ever feel confused about what to do in practice? Then use the framework in discussion with colleagues. Want to learn more about all this? Then we've given you some further reading to tap into.

Sounds confusing? Don't let it be! Listen, the majority of people go about their everyday lives using these ethical principles as a guide in making judgements, without necessarily even thinking about it. For many, these principles aren't really an issue in their working lives but, in nursing and midwifery, they're valuable in helping you make decisions ranging from staff rota organisation to ensuring patient care is effective and efficient, through to dealing with life-and-death emergency situations.

So let's put all of this information into practice. Consider the following scenarios and answer the questions at the end, jotting them down in your reflective diary.

⚠ ACTIVITY 10.4   CASE SCENARIOS

SCENARIO 1

Joe, a 74-year-old gentleman who's lived in a care home for about two years, is well liked by all the staff. One morning, Joe is being helped out of bed for his breakfast by staff who initially greet him and then start talking amongst themselves about their social events from the night before. As they help him into his wheelchair, Joe asks for his glasses but the staff don't hear him. As they wheel him out of the room into the dining area, Joe again asks for his glasses and again the staff don't hear him; they're too busy chatting. They transfer Joe to his table for breakfast where another member of staff greets him and asks what he'd like for breakfast from the menu. He tells her he hasn't got his glasses on – 'silly man' she replies, 'why did you forget them? Here's some porridge'. After about ten minutes, the carer returns and asks Joe why he hasn't eaten his porridge? He tells her that he's already said he needs his glasses to see properly before he can eat it. The carer then removes the porridge, which by now is cold, and leaves Joe looking at the table.

(Continued)

(Continued)

SCENARIO 2

Esme, a 24-year-old woman pregnant with her first baby, arrives at the maternity booking-in clinic with her partner. English isn't her first language and although she understands it, she doesn't speak very much and so lets her partner do the talking and translating for her. All appears to be going well until the midwife asks Esme for access to her arm to record her baseline blood pressure. There's a nervous look about Esme and her partner, who then tells her to remove her outer clothing for the midwife to gain access. At this point, the midwife notices a very large bruise on the upper part of Esme's arm, along with smaller ones below it. She asks Esme what happened and her partner replies that she's just silly and very clumsy; the bruise appeared after she'd tripped over and bumped into a cabinet. The midwife expresses concern and suggests Esme might want to spend the rest of the appointment with her in privacy without her partner. Esme looks at her partner and then shakes her head, indicating 'no'.

QUESTIONS TO PONDER:

1. What are the ethical issues that might arise from these scenario situations?
2. List the personal and professional values present in each situation – do they overlap?
3. How do these values and principles contribute to your dealing with these situations?

Want to learn more about similar situations to help you reflect on values, morals, ethics and safe practice? Then check out the NMC's safeguarding section and its associated DVD clips via the link here: www.nmc.org.uk/standards/safeguarding/training-toolkit/. While reflecting on these situations, you'll see that there are some complicated decisions to be made – decisions which could be adversely affected by your own personal values, that is, if you allow them to be made solely on the basis of your own opinions or beliefs. On the other hand though, if you apply the ethical principles of practice (as presented above), you can use these to question and guide your thoughts and actions to ensure the best outcome for your patient. And in doing that, don't forget that all patients have a right to be treated with dignity and respect as a unique individual in your care. This also means being aware of cultural differences; something else that can have an additional impact on ethical practice.

LEADERSHIP SKILLS

So far we've explored the key professional practice principles of accountability, honesty and integrity, and discussed the importance of acknowledging personal views, behaviour and attitudes as part of performance and ethical practice. As well as successfully completing a recognised and approved nursing or midwifery programme and achieving the specific competencies in your practice learning placements, the expectation is that, even as a student nurse or midwife, you'll apply the ethical principles of professional practice (NMC 2015a). By exploring and embedding these principles into your student life, you'll find you're better able to develop and refine them in your decision-making, and when prioritising care-related activities once qualified and registered.

But how does all of this relate to leadership in nursing and midwifery? Well, if you're aware of the above principles, you'll naturally begin to use them in your daily practice as a fully qualified and registered practitioner. You'll use your knowledge and understanding of people's individual situations to help you manage your time, decide upon your priorities and use the best available resources to meet their needs. Oh, and you'll sharpen your observation skills, assessment, evaluation and team-working abilities – those key leadership attributes that form part of your role as a nurse or midwife.

KEY RESPONSIBILITIES

While the NMC expects nurses and midwives to practice honestly and with integrity, using the best available evidence according to their roles and responsibilities, there are two overarching responsibilities which nurses and midwives must attain. One is revalidation (see Chapters 9 and 12) and the other is supervision. Although supervision is essential for both fields of practice, there are specific differences between nursing and midwifery.

In nursing, clinical supervision is achieved with colleagues in relation to everyday practice and often in response to specific, complex situations, whereas in midwifery, this is very different. Midwives are professionals in their own right, which means they've their own part of the NMC register and have specific standards for education and practice (NMC 2009), reflecting the independent role of the midwife (NMC 2012). These standards relate to every midwife working in the UK, whether working in the NHS, the private sector or self-employed. They must have an allocated supervisor of midwives – these are highly experienced midwives with additional training and education who guide midwives to develop their skills and expertise. They basically oversee the work of midwives on a regular basis to make sure they're meeting the high standards set by the profession. To be able to continue practising as a midwife, you'll need to complete an 'intention to practise' form and register this every year with your local supervising authority (NMC 2012). What about midwifery regulation? Check out 'Midwifery regulation' on the NMC website (www.nmc.org.uk/standards/what-to-expect-from-a-nurse-or-midwife/how-midwives-are-regulated/how-midwifery-regulation-works/).

Having been introduced to some of the key expectations and responsibilities in nursing and midwifery clinical practice, you'll now be in a stronger position to reflect and evaluate every clinical situation on its own merit, taking into account the patient's (and their family's) own individual situation. By becoming more aware of what makes you 'tick' and what your own values are, you'll be better placed to be more objective and take each situation on its own merit, using your skills of observation, assessment and clinical knowledge to plan and deliver non-judgemental care to meet the needs of patients. Being aware also of the specific responsibilities of supervision, especially in midwifery, should enable you to find out who your local supervisor of midwives is and how that relates to the role of the local supervising authority midwifery officer.

So, have we re-introduced you to those aspects of yourself which are inextricably linked to being a professional nurse or midwife? Have we helped you to examine your own values and behaviours? Have we helped you to appreciate how these link to the expectations placed upon you when you're delivering the key responsibilities of your professional role under the NMC Code (2015a)? We hope so! But it doesn't stop there. It's over to you now to practise what we've preached, to map out your professional career, and to continually professionally develop so that excellent patient care and service delivery become your professional mantra!

TOP TIPS

- ✔ Make a life size Buddy Billboard and write the key expectations of nursing or midwifery.
- ✔ Identify your personal values and moral beliefs and map these against the expectations.
- ✔ Read the Code, learn the Code, chunking three key rules at a time.
- ✔ Role play with peers a situation where your values are challenged – note your attitude and your approach.
- ✔ Use one clinical placement experience to reflect on your performance and note the positive and negative elements of this in your reflective diary.

So those are the tips, but don't forget your toolkit at the end of the book!

FURTHER READING 📖

Chief Nursing Officers of England, Northern Ireland, Scotland and Wales (2010) Midwifery 2020: Delivering Expectations. London: Department of Health (www. gov.uk/government/uploads/system/uploads/attachment_data/file/216029/ dh_119470.pdf).

Scrivener, R., Hand, T. and Hooper, R. (2011) 'Accountability and responsibility: principle of Nursing Practice B', *Nursing Standard*, 25(29): 35–36.

11 PLANNING AND PREPARING YOUR CAREER IN NURSING OR MIDWIFERY

⟹ So you want to work as a nurse or midwife?
⟹ Understanding your skills and how employers see you
⟹ Writing about yourself: CVs and applications
⟹ Talking about yourself: interviews and presentations
⟹ So what are your options after graduating?
⟹ Choosing your path
⟹ Changing your mind

CHAPTER OVERVIEW

As a student, it's easy to get caught up in the day-to-day activities of lectures, assignments and placements, while maintaining your social and family life. However, if you're to succeed in your career – whether you stay in nursing or midwifery or choose another professional path – you'll need to pause, reflect on your achievements, learn how to plan and choose your career path, and understand how to impress employers. This chapter shows you how to do just that by demonstrating your qualities and skills in your curriculum vitae (CV), applications and interviews so you land that dream job.

(Continued)

(Continued)

- So you want to work as a nurse or midwife?
- Understanding your skills and how employers see you
- Writing about yourself: CVs and applications

  o Covering letters
  o Writing successful job applications

- Talking about yourself: interviews and presentations
- So what are your options after graduating?
- Choosing your path

  o Overview of options

- Changing your mind
- Top tips

SO YOU WANT TO WORK AS A NURSE OR MIDWIFE?

You've completed your nursing or midwifery programme and you've acquired a lot of knowledge, skills and experience. So where to now? You've enjoyed this area, that area; you're interested in that speciality, this one – it's difficult to decide. Let's look back at what brought you into this profession – your motivation, your interests. Oh, and your goal – where you hoped to be once you qualified.

⛵ ACTIVITY 11.1   MOTIVATION, INTERESTS AND GOAL

So remind yourself of your motivation for coming into nursing or midwifery. Note it! Next note your specific interests and end goal. Now take that with you into your job search and interview, and you'll surely do well. Really want to impress? Then let's look at the skills you've developed along the way.

UNDERSTANDING YOUR SKILLS AND HOW EMPLOYERS SEE YOU

You come to your nursing and midwifery studies with specific qualities; they're yours – caring, compassionate, considerate – not something you learn but an innate part of who you are and what you stand for in life. As you develop, they also develop, becoming invaluable qualities for nursing and midwifery. But what about the skills you'll have heard discussed often in lectures or mentioned in practice placements?

Throughout your studies, you're encouraged to reflect on what you're learning so you understand where it fits into the overall framework of skills you'll need to work effectively as a nurse or midwife. So here are some of the key skills you'll hear about.

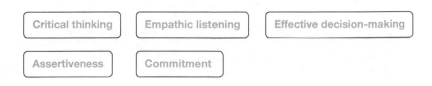

So how do you use these skills in the workplace?

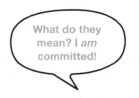

Sure you're committed. But are you fully committed to the lifelong learning evaluation of your personal and professional skills? That's what the NMC expect – come into the profession and the learning is for life. Why? Well, it's all about improving your practice in relation to patient care. And to do this you need to be conscientious about learning from the outset, exercise some critical thinking to help foster new knowledge and value evidence-based patient-care research. And when you're in the workplace, these skills should allow you to contribute to an ever-improving patient-care system where the skills you've learned become second-nature in your daily practice. So that's the few we've highlighted, but what about others? Can you think of other skills and learning you could talk about to an employer?

⚠️ **ACTIVITY 11.2   SKILLS FOR LIFE, SKILLS FOR EMPLOYERS**

Brainstorm with a group of friends and complete the framework in Table 11.1 to detail examples of how the NMC professional skills are applied in practice. What examples would you give an employer during a presentation for that dream job?

Table 11.1 Key transferable skills

Skills	Simple example	Detailed example
Effective listening	Receiving instruction from senior nurse	What is my role in the situation?
	Listening to a patient near the end of your shift	
	Discussion with a patient's family at the end of visiting hours	

You've surely learned these skills on your modules and practice learning placement, and understood their value – at least that's what your tutors hope is the case. You've maybe even started to apply them – at least that's what we hope you're learning to do; and that's what potential employers are hoping. So for a recap of the required professional skills, check out the NMC website for a comprehensive overview.

Still stuck for ideas? Why not look at your OAR? This should provide you with lots of detail about the activities you've covered and the learning your mentors say you've achieved at each stage of your course.

WRITING ABOUT YOURSELF: CVS AND APPLICATIONS

CV – our life on paper! So what do you need to know about me? How do I work out what's important to include and what's not so I land that job? What makes the perfect CV? Okay a few things to note:

- There's no such thing as a perfect CV and no strict rules as to what it should look like, so choose what works best for you.
- Employers tend to spend around 20 seconds doing an initial scan of a CV. The first page of this is where they're going to spend most of that time so that's where the most important information should go. If you put useful information, such as relevant experience, on the second page, it runs the risk of getting missed in this initial scan.
- Generic CVs are easy to spot and not as impressive as those tailored to a specific job. Be specific; different CV for different employers – show them exactly how you meet the criteria for their job, using the job description and any knowledge you may have about the particular role or workplace from placement.
- Your degree and your placement experiences particularly are likely to be key selling points in your CV. If you've any additional, relevant, employment history, such as from Bank work, then include that too.
- Different countries set different standards for CVs, so if you're planning to work abroad check the required standards: some employers prefer a one-page résumé rather than a two-page CV. Get it right from the outset!

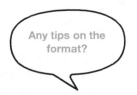

Any tips on the format?

Sure, your CV needs to be logical, clear, concise and in an accessible format. While there are three main types – chronological, skills-based, and a combination of the two – the chronological is by far the most popular (see www.rcn.org.uk/professional-develop ment/find-a-job/cv-writing for an example). The following pointers will ensure a clear presentation:

- Two A4 sides.
- Sans serif font, e.g. Arial, 12 point.
- Font styles, e.g. bold – only use for headings or when highlighting important information, such as your degree title.

- Use short paragraphs and bullet points to help the reader find information more readily.
- Use professional language when describing your skills and experience. Get your message across; use positive action words such as managed, co-ordinated.
- Spelling and grammar – get it proofread by a person or use specialist software.

> What if I've a lot of previous employment?

Remember, stick to the concise format and summarise your experience, for example, 'four years' experience in social care services'. Alternatively, simply list your job titles, employers and employment dates.

> What if I've no relevant previous employment?

While it's always an advantage to have some relevant previous employment, students and new graduates aren't expected to have much experience, other than what they've done on placement. Even so, it's possible to use information from your studies to demonstrate your knowledge and skills, such as project work in a specific area. Transferable skills from previous employment or positions of responsibility are also important.

> What if there's a gap in my employment history?

You never know how an employer will view your CV – close inspection of employment history versus recently acquired, relevant skills – so always explain the gaps. You can do this here or briefly in your covering letter. Using the chronological format? Then provide a brief explanation beside each gap, for example, '2006–2012: full-time care commitments'. If the gap requires more explanation, then briefly discuss this in your covering letter.

> What about including a personal statement in my CV?

Personal statements are generally optional and usually sit at the top of your CV. Want to highlight your key selling points for a particular job, for example, 'experience of working with vulnerable people' when applying for a job in a care home for the elderly? Then include a personal statement. Don't include one if you're writing a general statement that doesn't really give much added value to your CV, for example, 'can work independently or as part of a team'. That's the CV, now here's the covering letter.

COVERING LETTERS

Okay, I've received your application for the post and am about to read your covering letter, so what have you told me? I hope it's interesting as this is my first introduction to you. Have you impressed me? I hope so; otherwise, I won't want to read your CV!

> This is my first ever covering letter; can you give me a few tips then?

Here you go:

- Don't send generic covering letters; they're easy to spot and don't impress employers!
- Always tailor your covering letter to suit individual employers and jobs.
- If you're sending an emailed application the body of your email often becomes your covering letter, in which case you don't need to follow the standard business letter layout.
- In emailed applications, write professionally, use a capital letter for the pronoun 'I', and don't use text language or emoticons.
- If you're sending the letter to a named person then you can sign off the letter 'Yours sincerely'. If not, then address the recipient 'Dear Sir/Madam' and sign off as 'Yours faithfully'. If using email then signing off with 'Regards' is acceptable.
- Start your letter by stating which job you're applying for, including its reference number (if there is one), and mention where the job was advertised.
- Close the letter by thanking the employer for considering your application.

Although there are no rules as to the order of the rest of the letter, it's important you include the following:

- Why you're interested in this organisation and, in particular, this specific job. While this can be the most difficult part to write, it's the piece that can make your letter stand out. Let them see that you've done your research, know who they are and investigated the job specifics, then show how the information you've discovered fits with your interests and career plans. Whatever you do, don't copy and paste from their website. That doesn't impress!
- Summarise how you meet the criteria the employer is looking for, what you can bring to the organisation and the job specifically, and highlight any key or transferable skills or knowledge you can use in this specific role. Refer the reader to your CV for further details.
- Keep the letter to one A4 page.

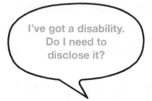

I've got a disability. Do I need to disclose it?

Well, I'd say it's probably best to do so, even though there's no legal requirement to disclose a disability to an employer in your CV or covering letter. Look at the positives though:

- It helps to highlight personal strengths.
- It improves your access to equal opportunities and training schemes.
- It raises awareness of any additional support you might require in the recruitment process to even out the field.

Disclosing in your covering letter? Then focus on the positive. Tell them what you can do rather than what you can't, discuss your skills and strengths and the different perspective these can offer their organisation.

What if I've a criminal record? Should I disclose?

Nurses are held to a higher standard than many other professions. The NMC Code (2015a) makes it clear that you must disclose to both the NMC and your current or potential employer as soon as you can: '... any caution or charge against you, or if you have received a conditional discharge in relation to, or have been found guilty of a criminal offence (other than a protected caution or conviction)' (paragraph 23.2).

If you're unsure if your offence is a protected one, follow the NMC guidance (www.nmc.org.uk/registration/staying-on-the-register/

informing-us-of-cautions-and-convictions/). This also applies to the revalidation process, and, if you're still a student, you must inform your university of any new or pending criminal convictions.

WRITING SUCCESSFUL JOB APPLICATIONS

Want to land your dream job? Then let's start with some basic principles of the successful job application and some useful specifics for NHS applications. Remember, the application form is usually the first stage of an employer's recruitment process and the point when most applicants are rejected. So, want to improve your chances of progressing to the next stage? Then avoid those simple, common mistakes:

- Answer all of the questions on the form, providing as much detail as possible.
- Don't write 'see attached CV' to answer any question.
- Whatever you do, don't get rejected because of a small spelling or grammatical error. Get your form proofread or run it through an online spellchecker.
- Some professional applications can take a long time to complete so don't rush through yours. Want that job? Then consider your answers and the information you provide.
- Completing an online application form? Then note your password.

Application complete? Need reassurance that it all looks good before submitting? Then ask your Careers Adviser to check it. After all, understanding job applications is their job, is it not?

Okay that's my application form, but what about my personal statement? I need to tell them how I'm right for this job; how do I actually do that?

Okay, let's see. It's your statement and it's personal to you but that doesn't always make it easy to write. A few pointers then:

- Read the job description carefully and jot down the criteria the employer is looking for.
- Start by explaining why you're applying for this specific job; what you find interesting about it.
- Briefly tell them the qualities you feel you can bring to it.
- Describe how you meet the criteria and give some examples to support this.
- Not quite sure what they expect in an application? Then check out the Royal College of Nursing website (www.rcn.org.uk/pro fessional-development/find-a-job/cv-writing) for some examples.

⚠ ACTIVITY 11.3   WHO ARE YOU REALLY?

Struggling to write about yourself? Then work with a friend; they know you and your qualities – scribble them on post-its and put them on your Buddy Billboard, noting why this quality is important and valuable for this job.

> What if I get asked competency questions in my application? What are they exactly and how would I deal with them?

They're questions that typically begin with 'Give me an example of a time when ...' or 'Describe a time ...'. Don't forget you're likely to encounter these types of question at interview also. So two tips:

1. Give your examples from something familiar – your study, part-time work, hobbies and interests.
2. Use the STAR technique (S = Situation, T = Task, A = Action, R = Result) to format your answers (www.gradjobs.co.uk/careers-

advice/interview-advice/using-the-star-technique-to-succeed-at-interviews). Allocate equal amounts of attention to the Situation and Action parts of your answer.

That's your application, now what about your interview.

TALKING ABOUT YOURSELF: INTERVIEWS AND PRESENTATIONS

Well, I've read all about you on paper. Now tell me who you really are and why I should offer you this job and not the next person. Want this job? Then before I interview you, I'll expect you to:

- Check out the organisation's website to find more out about both the organisation and the role you're applying for.
- Check out www.glassdoor.co.uk/ to see what it's like working for the organisation from the employee's perspective.
- Know the logistics of how to get to your interview location, plan the route, time the route and build in extra time for any diversions or unexpected happenings.
- Know the interview format; does it contain a presentation? If so, then recap on managing your presentation (see Chapter 6).
- Understand the importance of body language and the need to create a positive first impression (see Appendix 7 for links).
- Practise common interview questions (see Appendix 7 for links).

Remember, interview questions typically fall into one of the following categories:

- You and your motivation for applying for the job.
- Your understanding of the role and the organisation.
- How you behave and interact with others (often competency questions which employers expect to be answered in the STAR format mentioned above).

So prepare your examples before the interview; don't get caught out trying to come up with some on the spot. Take care to maintain patient confidentiality (NMC 2015a) when considering your examples – no names please! Want to find out more about the organisation? Then think of some questions you could ask once you've researched a little about them. Remember, these should be questions you'd have difficulty finding the answer to before your interview.

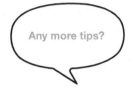

Any more tips?

Sure, check out interview information on the following websites: Prospects, Targetjobs, Graduate Recruitment Bureau, Wikijob, and Best job interview (Appendix 7). Some sites cover general interviews while others are more specifically targeted at student and graduate interviews.

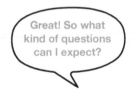

Great! So what kind of questions can I expect?

Okay, let's see:

Q: Talk us through an example that demonstrates your ability to deal effectively with emergency situations.

Q: Describe a time when you used your communication skills to improve the care of one of your patients.

Q: Describe a situation when you used your leadership skills to resolve a difficult patient situation.

Q: Tell us about a change you made (or observed) in working practice to improve patient safety.

Q: How would you go about ensuring that you improve your patient's quality of care?

Q: Tell us about a decision you made recently that had a positive effect on your patient's care.

Q: A family believe that your community-based patient is at risk – how do you assess this?

Q: There's aggression between two patients on a ward – how do you deal with it?

Q: What approaches should be used to reduce the incidence of violence?

Enough? That should give you an idea of what you could be asked. Why not practise with your peers; help each other along, give feedback. Better still, arrange a mock interview with your Careers Adviser; this should allay your interview fears.

SO WHAT ARE YOUR OPTIONS AFTER GRADUATING?

Well I've graduated now so I guess I need to start looking for a job. Any good tips for me?

Sure, here are five things to remember when job seeking:

1. Systematically note every job you're applying for, as well as what stage you're at with each application. If your application stops at the written application stage, ask for feedback. Feedback is helpful for future applications so you know why you've not made it to interview. But note, not all employers automatically provide feedback at this stage, so if you want feedback to feed forward then ask! Made it to interview but

didn't get the job? Then ask for feedback on your interview performance so you can improve your interview skills.

2. Check out the various careers websites (Appendix 7); get a feel for those that have jobs you can realistically apply for at this stage. Don't want to miss something interesting? Then set up job alerts and don't forget to regularly check in on your favourite sites. You never know, your dream job might just be there!

3. Motivation! Know yours! Understand why you're applying for a particular job. What attracts you? Do you know the workplace already? Can you afford to live in the area? Does the vacancy provide the right level of learning opportunities you need at this stage in your career? With the right level of motivation, you'll shine through at both application and interview stage, so know yours!

4. Take time not to waste time! Treat every application seriously – after all you want that job. Yes? Then don't submit a weak application. If you do, you're only wasting time – yours and your potential employer's. So carefully consider the questions and why you're applying for this particular job. Remember motivation!

5. Need some advice and inspiration to improve and strengthen your application before submitting it? Then draw on the experience of others – peers, PDT/DoS, placement colleagues and mentor, and your university careers adviser.

So those are the tips, now for the job search. Although the majority of UK nursing and midwifery vacancies are within the NHS, the public and private sectors, medical charities and armed forces, amongst others, also offer a range of opportunities (Appendix 7). Specialist nursing agencies also recruit for both permanent and temporary positions at home and abroad (Appendix 7).

I'd like to work in Ireland, but I trained in the UK. Is there anything specific I need to do to practise there?

You'll find all you need to know in the nurses and midwives guide at the Nursing and Midwifery Board of Ireland website (Appendix 7). The Board also provides full guidance on Irish careers options for nurses and midwives at Nursing Careers (Appendix 7).

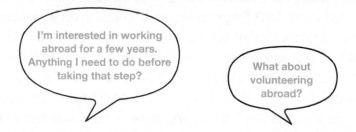

I'm interested in working abroad for a few years. Anything I need to do before taking that step?

What about volunteering abroad?

Although some graduates move overseas immediately following graduation, most prefer to remain in the UK to consolidate their training and gain some solid experience in their specific field. With that behind them, they're in a stronger position to compete for good overseas opportunities. So when you get those restless feet for something new, somewhere new, start searching the RCN, RCM, Prospects and Going Global websites for information on working abroad (Appendix 7). The NMC also has a whole section of its website devoted to working outside the UK, including how to register with the relevant overseas authority (Appendix 7).

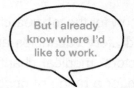

But I already know where I'd like to work.

Well in that case, identify the relevant nursing authority for that country and check out their guidance so your journey and employment there goes without a hiccup (Appendix 7).

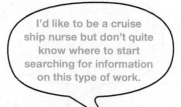

I'd like to be a cruise ship nurse but don't quite know where to start searching for information on this type of work.

You'll find all you need to know in a few websites – Cruise Ship Medical Jobs, All Cruise Jobs and Redgoldfish (Appendix 7). While cruise ship work sounds 'romantic', be aware that you'll be on call 24/7. Working alongside a team of other medical professionals, you'll provide both routine and emergency treatments, so it's helpful to have some Accident and Emergency experience under your belt.

CHOOSING YOUR PATH

Nursing and midwifery qualifications are your passport to different branches of nursing or midwifery, diverse specialities and the doorway to a whole host of other healthcare professions with a variety of people in a range of settings. Building on your basic qualification, you can continue with shortened courses, accelerated second undergraduate courses or postgraduate courses to give you the knowledge and expertise you need for that dream job. Note the pathway though! While accelerated nursing degrees are open to all graduates regardless of their subject area, the shortened midwifery course is available only to registered nurses, and not in all universities. So check out where you're thinking of studying for more information. Feel some examples would be useful? Then check out Appendix 7 for:

- NHS Careers – a website aimed at pre-registered nurses and midwives containing video case studies featuring careers from different areas.
- Prospects: Options with Nursing – gives you insight into the skills you gain on a nursing degree, as well as the job options available to you on registration.
- Just for Nurses – provides an array of professional articles, discussion forum and jobs boards.

From all fields of nursing practice and midwifery, you'll find a range of employment opportunities both within and outside the NHS – working in acute hospital and community settings, providing care across an integrated health and social care service. Midwives will generally work within the NHS or private sectors across acute and community settings.

OVERVIEW OF OPTIONS

So you want to be a nurse or a midwife? You walked through the university doors to start your studies. You've been on many different placements and have an idea of the area you'd like to work in but wouldn't you like to know all the options? Be aware – some areas require additional qualifications and experience, but don't let that put you off. Go on – keep the goal in mind!

Okay, for more specifics about the options available in the different disciplines and the various settings see Appendix 8, but remember, these lists aren't exhaustive and don't contain every single job available for these fields of practice. They're simply a taster of what's out there! Oh, and note, depending on the area you choose to work in, the posts will be tailored to meet the needs of the local population; not all job types are available in every area.

So that gives you a flavour of the different jobs out there. None of them appeal? Considering something else? Not sure what? Well, here are a few tips.

CHANGING YOUR MIND

So nursing or midwifery isn't quite 'hitting the spot' for you? You'd prefer something more, even different? How about occupational therapy, speech and language therapy, physiotherapy, dietetics? Oh no, more study, I hear you say. Sure, but it's on an accelerated graduate entry route, so shorter! Think of the added value you'll bring to these allied health professions with your nursing and/or midwifery knowledge and experience. Or how about social work, youth or community work, medical sales or lecturing?

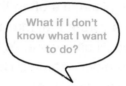

Your practice learning placements ideally should give you an idea of the area you'd like to work in but if you've completed your degree and are still wondering, then don't worry. We've all been there; it's not so unusual, you know. Talk to others, what's their experience, ask for advice and check out the options again on the NHS Careers and Prospects websites. Who knows, you might fall into something that's not directly related to your degree; something you might never have thought of but which fits your skills and personality perfectly. So with a little help, you'll get there. We all do!

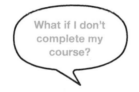

Sometimes things don't work out as we expected. We've struggled with the academic work, we can't afford to study any more, or quite simply nursing or midwifery just doesn't match up. Leaving is the only option. But before you make that decision chat to family and friends to help you make sure you're absolutely sure about leaving. Feel some professional advice would be helpful to make sure you understand all the options? Then tap into your SSFA (Chapter 2) – chat to your careers adviser, student counsellor or PDT/DoS. Perhaps some time out will help you in your decision to leave permanently and pursue another career. Ideally it might not be what you want but in the long run it's sure to work out for the best. Many graduates have done this and ended up successfully working in an area not directly related to their degree, for example, Allied Health, Education or Social Work.

No matter what your final decision is regarding your place of work, remember that the first post you take on after qualifying is where the 'real' learning takes place. It's often the first step on the rung of your career ladder – a career that may take you in lots of different directions, where you'll gain valuable knowledge and skills to work across health and other settings. No matter what happens, use this first stage of employment as your 'grounding' or 'consolidating' opportunity. A time when you'll put all you've learned at university and in placement into practice.

Remember, practice makes perfect; as you gain experience you'll also gain confidence to open up your thoughts to different areas of nursing and midwifery. Some of this might involve further study, some not – but whatever you do, know it will also be exciting, challenging and most worthwhile.

TOP TIPS

- ✔ Use shaped post-its to shape your career path – write your motivation, interests, goals, options.
- ✔ Reflect on your choices and how your skills can be best used, and note them in your journal.
- ✔ Practise your presentations skills with your friends or peers.
- ✔ Hold a peer supported workshop on 'your qualities and skills'.
- ✔ Do mock interviews with your Careers Adviser.
- ✔ Practise writing covering letters, CVs, and your personal statement, and get feedback from your peers or Careers Adviser.
- ✔ Keep a mind map or spreadsheet of your job applications, and a timeline of what stage they're at.
- ✔ Research potential employers and organisations and keep an alphabetical folder for future reference.

So those are the tips, but don't forget your toolkit at the end of the book!

FURTHER READING

Borrego, M. and Bird, J. (2010) *Careers Uncovered: Nursing and Midwifery.* Surrey: Trotman Publishing.
Smoker, A. (2016) *Launching Your Career in Nursing and Midwifery: A Practical Guide.* London: Palgrave.

12 DEVELOPING YOUR PROFESSIONALISM

- Continuing professional development – what it means and who it's for
- Keeping up to date – whose responsibility?
- Keep up to date; keep up to scratch – but where do you start?
- Why join a union?
- Maintaining and retaining your professional registration
- Taking a career break – maternity leave or other leave of absence

 CHAPTER OVERVIEW

You're living through a time of great change. All over the world, new technologies and techniques are transforming people's lives and their expectations of what they can achieve in life. For nurses and midwives, this means you're better able to care for your patients thanks to greater knowledge and sharing of good practice by your fellow professionals. However, patients' higher expectations bring with them greater scrutiny of you as a professional, and of your ability to give them the very best available care. To help you live up to these expectations, this chapter explores the importance of developing and maintaining your professionalism and discusses how this will benefit your practice and your career; giving you tips on how to keep on top of things along the way.

- Continuing professional development – what it means and who it's for
- Keeping up to date – whose responsibility?
- Keep up to date; keep up to scratch – but where do you start?

    o So what's on offer?

(Continued)

CONTINUING PROFESSIONAL DEVELOPMENT – WHAT IT MEANS AND WHO IT'S FOR

Continuing professional development (CPD) is what you do to maintain the skills and knowledge required to do your job successfully throughout your professional life. If you thought most of your learning would stop after finishing university – think again! Don't worry though, most professionals say they really enjoy CPD and would like more of it so they can become the best nurse or midwife they can be. So who's CPD for then? Well, in short – you!

CPD is defined by the Health & Care Professions Council (HCPC) (2015) as 'a range of learning activities through which health and care professionals maintain and develop throughout their career to ensure that they retain their capacity to practise safely, effectively and legally within their evolving scope of practice' (www. hpc-uk.org/aboutregistration/standards/cpd/).

The Code (NMC 2015a) states that CPD is a vital activity for nurses and midwives to improve practice, to learn and develop throughout their careers, and to keep their skills and knowledge up to date, to enable them to work safely, legally and effectively.

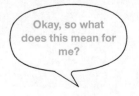

Okay, so what does this mean for me?

Well, five things really. It means that:

- You begin your career knowing you're entering a profession where you'll never stop learning new things, and where you'll be expected to keep learning and demonstrate that learning.
- You'll need to find employers willing to invest in you and keep you at the forefront of your profession, so you're able to give the best possible care.
- You'll need to consider how to develop beyond your current job requirements, if you're to achieve promotion or seniority with your own employer, or even compete for a job elsewhere.
- You'll always need to be doing enough and learning enough to retain your professional registration, even if you cut your hours or take time out for whatever reason.
- You'll need to record and reflect on your own achievements and skills by completing your professional portfolio (Andre and Heartfield 2011).

This sounds like a lot of hard work I know, but nurses and midwives are used to that. Besides, we're giving you this handbook to make being professional a lot easier!

KEEPING UP TO DATE – WHOSE RESPONSIBILITY?

As a student, you'll receive lots of help and support so you can learn effectively. You'll be given the tools, but, at the end of the day, it's your responsibility to make the most of what's on offer, so you can achieve the required standard to pass your modules and placements – oh, and ultimately gain your degree. Working life, well that's no different – you're ultimately responsible for your own work. In nursing and midwifery though, there's also a formal recognition that your employer must support you, so you can achieve and maintain your professional standards. The formal standards and regulations of the NMC (2012; 2014) dictate what's required for you to be recognised as a professional nurse or midwife. These are the same standards and regulations your employer refers to when asking you to undertake workplace duties. Ultimately though, it's entirely your professional responsibility to ensure you're providing appropriate care. So keep up to date! Want your patients to be confident in your professionalism? Then do what it takes to maintain your registration and get revalidated every three years (NMC 2015c).

Put yourself in their shoes – as a potential patient yourself, I'm sure you'd expect nothing less than to be cared for by someone who's fully qualified with proven skills. So place The Code (NMC 2015a) at the heart of all you do and you'll surely achieve those high standards and ensure you're up to date and fit to practise (see Chapter 10). Let's see, you've passed your degree, you've consolidated your skills and learning, and you've secured a suitable post. So how can you improve and develop your skills?

A good employer will have a system in place to ensure that all of their employees have the right training and qualifications, or can at least work towards them. In the UK, each NHS post has specific dimensions or responsibilities known as the Knowledge Skills Framework (KSF), which all staff have to achieve (www.ksf. scot.nhs.uk/; www.nhsemployers.org/SimplifiedKSF). The KSF aims to support a consistent approach to personal development planning (PDP) where its key dimensions function as a base in regular reviews with your manager to ensure you're achieving the key requirements of your post. Even if your employer doesn't use this system, the framework can be a useful basis for discussion of your development.

Want to consider ways of developing your skills so you can enhance your patient care? Want to meet the overall needs of your particular employer and be fit to practise? You do! Then plan your career and future study! Be open to ideas and your employer's encouragement, explore new ways of working, and be all you can be as a professional.

KEEP UP TO DATE; KEEP UP TO SCRATCH – BUT WHERE DO YOU START?

Well, I guess the best place to start is seeing how you measure up to the four key domains outlined in the NMC Code (2015a).

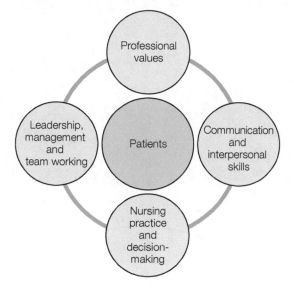

Figure 12.1   NMC four domains

So let's look at one section of The Code to see how you're measuring up.

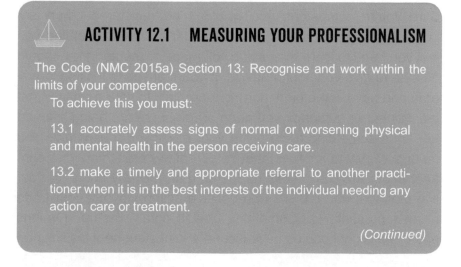

ACTIVITY 12.1   MEASURING YOUR PROFESSIONALISM

The Code (NMC 2015a) Section 13: Recognise and work within the limits of your competence.
    To achieve this you must:

13.1 accurately assess signs of normal or worsening physical and mental health in the person receiving care.

13.2 make a timely and appropriate referral to another practitioner when it is in the best interests of the individual needing any action, care or treatment.

(Continued)

(Continued)

13.3 ask for help from a suitably qualified and experienced healthcare professional to carry out any action or procedure that is beyond the limits of your competence.

13.4 take account of your own personal safety as well as the safety of people in your care, and,

13.5 complete the necessary training before carrying out a new role.

So let's scale how you meet these standards; circle your answer

Exceptional   Good   Acceptable   Poor

Now note any areas where you're feeling unsure or under-trained.

Oh no – it's a long list! I don't feel very competent now when I look at that.

Sure you're competent; you wouldn't be registered otherwise. Look at this list as your friend! If it's just a small something you feel you need to learn then ask a colleague or mentor; they should be able to give you sound advice. If you feel you're lacking in any area and have something more to learn, talk to your manager; get the training or guidance you need. Feel you're not being listened to? Then something to note – if your employer doesn't give you an opportunity to improve, they're potentially breaching your contract under the KSF. If this happens, then formally speak to your line manager and if there's no positive action, contact your trade union representative. Something else to note – the trade unions and professional bodies have issued a joint statement insisting on a minimum of six days/45 hours paid time off per year of CPD for all healthcare professionals, with adequate staffing replacement to ensure patient care isn't adversely affected when you're off. Not only will your employer be aware of this but they should be facilitating this for you. Remember, the NMC revalidation process requires you to have a minimum level of CPD. So that's for you to note!

Want to see how you measure up against all sections of the Code? Then either repeat Activity 12.1 across the Code or use your employer's personal appraisal/review documents (Appendix 9) to highlight any areas of development or improvement. Note it and take charge of your own career development!

SO WHAT'S ON OFFER?

> Okay, so actually doing the training and keeping my knowledge up to date; how does that work then?

Well, even though you're learning a lot on the job from colleagues, you're still required to reflect on this and record it all for revalidation purposes. Your employer is likely to be key to any further formal training you receive. They'll normally be plugged into training networks provided by your fellow professionals or academic specialists, and they'll normally contribute to the cost of your training, either with time as study leave (letting you undertake the study during work time) or by paying for the course or training. Sounds great! But note – they don't always do both, which means you'll need to take some ownership of your own CPD requirements.

Anything else on offer? Well, sometimes in-house training is provided; for example, where a visiting trainer offers a CPD session on a specific area with a group of your colleagues. Then again, there are the NHS coordinated networks; maybe there's one in your city or region? Want to check out an example? Then click the link for the 2016 Scottish Multi-professional Maternity Development Programme (www.scottishmaternity.org/). Here you'll find training events on offer at different Scottish maternity hospitals on a wide range of practical topics, from neonatal resuscitation to routine examination of newborns. There's also the National Managed Network Service (NMNS) and the Strategic Clinical Networks Service providing a whole range of information relating to different specialities (see Appendix 9 for links).

Find this interesting? Then speak to your employer first about attending such courses to make sure they're in line with your professional development needs. Who knows, your CPD training may well find you back at your old university or one nearby in future – doing either a short course on something like taking blood, or even a post-degree top up or Masters. Want to progress to a more specialist, senior or leadership role? Then it's likely you'll need to achieve further qualifications. An increasing emphasis is also being placed on doing research, with support available for the development of clinical research careers across the UK – check out your local university or local clinical research office. So, want to know more about potential training possibilities relevant to your own needs or wishes? Then speak to the person responsible for your training at work, or seek advice from lecturing staff at your old university, or even from your trade union contacts.

So, you walked through the university doors; you stayed 'on course'; you completed your programme; and you qualified and registered. And all along, you'd an idea of the area you wanted to specialise and work in, then something changed. Something that wasn't quite clear to you when you'd started but which caught your interest over time.

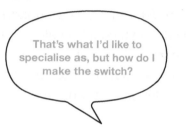

Well, you may not receive training just because you want it! So be prepared to be determined; justify your choices, make your employer aware of the mutual practical benefits of supporting you to develop and learn more about this area of practice. Why not use the SMART technique to justify your request (see Appendix 10). A key tip here is to link any study opportunities to your current role – that way your employers can't argue with it! After all, it's your career, it's your future, and it's your responsibility to make it all happen!

WHY JOIN A UNION?

Well why not? Most nurses and midwives working in the NHS or other public sector employers are lucky enough to be in a position to join one of the recognised unions – the RCM, RCN or UNISON (see Appendix 9). Good employers are always happy to recommend that you join a trade union; this makes it easier for them to consult with you on a whole variety of things. Oh, and there's the advantage of having a unified voice when trying to negotiate or improve your pay and conditions, not to mention your professional standing. Great! Anything else?

Sure, unions everywhere can help in times of trouble, for example, when you've issues with sickness or stress, or face disciplinary action. Importantly, they'll also represent you when faced with questions relating to your professional conduct, or following a complaint or legal challenge involving you. This can be a complex and worrying process, so it's worth having the right expert support when you need it most. The support doesn't stop there. Unions produce written materials to help you learn and develop in your professional career. For example, guides on issues relating to your professional revalidation or to your agreed training opportunities. So there's a lot on offer and a lot of benefits from joining the Union.

> But I'm still a student.

Doesn't matter. Best time to join the union! Join as a student and you'll get access to special offers on books or journals. Think of the savings! So make full use of the resources that can help you both as a student and for professional development purposes.

MAINTAINING AND RETAINING YOUR PROFESSIONAL REGISTRATION

So you've registered with the NMC but how do you actually maintain and retain this? Simple! You need to maintain so you can retain! Maintain it by keeping up to date and meeting the 'fit to practise' criteria; retain it by revalidating your registration every three years. Want to continue practising? Then revalidation is essential; it's your responsibility remember. Want to demonstrate your continued ability to practise safely and effectively? Then look at it as a positive process and not as something that challenges your fitness to practise; any concerns about this are dealt with differently. So boost your levels of professionalism; remember to keep a reflective diary, think about your career development and provide evidence about what you do on a daily basis in practice.

WHAT'S REVALIDATION?

Well, it's something all nurses and midwives in the UK need to undertake every three years to maintain their registration. It's a process where you're able to squarely reflect on the role of the NMC Code (2015a) in your practice, and show that you're a safe and efficient practitioner who maintains the professional standards and competencies. Revalidation is more about promoting good practice across the profession than it is measuring your fitness to practise. So look back at Chapter 10 to see your revalidation obligations.

Something to note – maintaining and retaining, professionally developing and revalidating are all things you'll be engaging with for the rest of your career. Oh yes! Just think though, it should be much easier for you than for your more experienced colleagues; you've had lots more recent experience of recording your work and reflecting on your development needs. So be a good colleague – share your enthusiasm, demonstrate your professionalism, share good practice and draw on your colleagues' revalidation wisdom! Think of the mutual benefits!

Something else to note – while the revalidation process lets you ask for training in line with the NMC Code (2015a), it's also designed to fit in with your employer's standard appraisal/review systems.

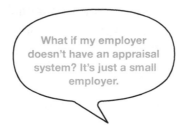

What if my employer doesn't have an appraisal system? It's just a small employer.

Well, if you're registered with the NMC as a nurse or midwife, your employer has a duty to help you maintain your registration and keep up to date with professional advances relevant to your post.

Ask them what their procedures are for staff appraisal/review and familiarise yourself with the paperwork.

TAKING A CAREER BREAK – MATERNITY LEAVE OR OTHER LEAVE OF ABSENCE

Sometimes life dictates your need for a career break; it's not unusual. People take breaks for a variety of reasons. Don't forget though to maintain your registration as a nurse or midwife, you'll need to meet the current minimum practice requirements of 450 hours over a pre-break three-year period, or 900 hours if maintaining registration for both professions (see NMC guidance for full details). But if you can't meet this requirement, it's worth knowing your options:

> You can successfully complete an appropriate NMC approved return to practice programme before the date of your revalidation application. These programmes are designed to allow you to renew your registration and return to practice after a break in practice. You can cancel your registration. You will continue to hold a nursing or midwifery qualification, but will not be a registered nurse or midwife. You can apply for readmission to the register in future, if you wish to practise as a nurse or midwife. (NMC 2015c: 14.33)

So let's recap – revalidation is an essential requirement for all nurses and midwives and needs to be done in particular ways. If you simply follow the NMC guidance and work with your employer, you'll achieve the desired result.

Here are a few key things to remember:

1. Feedback: it's important – whether formal, informal, written, verbal, relating to you or your team – and you'll get this from patients, colleagues, trainers, teachers, reports or through your formal appraisals. So consider how it relates to you

personally and how you can feed it forward to develop your skills and knowledge. Keep a record of it! As with your assignment feedback, you'll feel it's not always positive but don't take it personally. Look at it as something supportive, where you can learn from the constructive criticism.

2. Portfolio: whether electronic or written, record and store up-to-date evidence of your practice; that's important too (Andre and Heartfield 2011). Again, refer to the NMC guidance.

Seems straightforward enough on paper but in practice, mmm – maybe you need help with the revalidation process because of a particular difficulty like dyslexia. Then why not start preparing early and contact the NMC for advice. Don't worry though, your employer should be able to support you here. If they can't or won't, then speak to your trade union. They're sure to offer help.

So that's it – from graduation to registration, to maintaining and retaining, professionally developing and revalidating – it's a lot of work I know, but think of the opportunity to improve your skills, learn more about yourself and others, and develop your career. So make the most of it! Go on, you know you want to!

TOP TIPS

✓ Keep a CPD journal – record your CPD activities in a hard copy notebook, a 5-year diary or electronic portfolio (see NMC revalidation section for an example). Keep this in addition to any formal paperwork you receive from your employer. It will help you to have a proper perspective on your overall development, not simply what your current employer wants from you.

✓ Be SMART (Specific, Measurable, Action-focused, Realistic, Time-bound). Set yourself goals to achieve in the short, medium and long term (see Appendix 10 for example).

✓ Be a SWOT – look at your Strengths (both personal and professional), Weaknesses (both personal and professional), Opportunities (for your learning) and Threats (things that get in the way of your learning).

(Continued)

(Continued)

✓ Do a SWOT analysis of where you're at now in your current job.
✓ Repeat the SWOT analysis at every stage of your professional career.
✓ Regularly review your situation and reassess your skills.
✓ Attend training and events programmes.
✓ Actively seek out any available training.
✓ Keep a note of courses that interest you.
✓ Make a date to undertake the training.
✓ Complete your CPD journal following training.
✓ Ask the right questions of your fellow professionals, both about their work, and any training and development opportunities.
✓ Listen to colleagues' views on how to practise effectively, and the training opportunities they found most useful.
✓ Observe good practice and explore training possibilities.

So those are the tips, but don't forget your toolkit at the end of the book!

FURTHER READING

Coombs, J. (2015) *Nurses Reflective Diary: Revalidation.* Colorado Springs: Create Space Independent Publishing Platform.

Davies, P. (2013) *How to Get Through Revalidation: Making the Process Easy.* Boca Raton, FL: CRC Press.

NMC Revalidation: http://revalidation.nmc.org.uk/welcome-to-revalidation

YOUR NURSING AND MIDWIFERY TOOLKIT

We all need to learn how to reflect on what we do so we can do things differently and maybe even better next time around, helping us to become a more effective learner and a more focused, evolving professional practitioner. To help you achieve that, we've pulled together a range of tools to support your learning. You should find something here that suits your learning style and works for you.

Visual Tools

- Map it …
- Colour it …
- Picture it …
- Shape it …

Colour it …
Coloured Stickers
Doodle Pad
Shaped Post-Its
ShiftHub

Picture it …
Flashcards
Medincle
NMC DVD clips
Storyboard
Videoscribe
Whiteboard

Map it …
Bubbl.us
Buddy Billboard
Claro Software
Inspiration Software
Juggling Man
Mapping Man
Note Nuggets
Presentation Pyramid
Wisemapping

Shape it …
5Rs assessment wheel
GapMap Bridge
Stop, Start, Improve, Consider
Student Support First Aider Heart
Thought Pot

Auditory Tools

Read it …
- Careers-related websites – NMC, RCN, RC
- Dictionary
- Equality Act/Disability-related legislation
- Feedback notes
- NMC revalidation booklet
- Medical Dictionary
- NICE Guidance
- NMC Code
- NMC Record Keeping Guidance
- NMC Social Media Guidance
- Primary Maths book
- Student Charters – NMC/University
- The Little Book of Procrastination
- University online money guide

Attend it …
- Careers-related workshops – CV, completing applications, cover letters, mock interviews
- Skills workshops – Giving Presentations, Communication Skills, Confidence Building, Being Assertive, Knowing yourself and your skills

Hear it … / **Use it …**
- Apps – relaxation, student support
- Language Line
- Mentors and Peers
- Moodle discussion room
- Podcasts
- Relaxation music
- YouTube
- Drug Calculation Manual
- Evidently Cochrane
- Facebook
- Library resources
- NHS Open Athens
- Out of hours services – NHS 24,
- Samaritans, Breathing Space,
- Mind, Penumbra
- Peer support network
- Portable Harvard Reference app
- RCN/RCM website – latest news and research
- Snapchat
- SSFA Advisers
- Study Buddy
- Thesaurus
- Trade Union
- Translation App
- Turnitin
- Twitter
- Your eyes, ears and mouth!

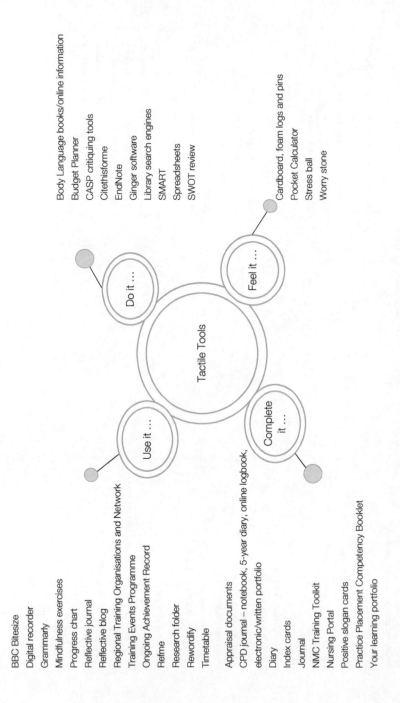

Tactile Tools

Do it ...

Use it ...

Feel it ...

Complete it ...

Body Language books/online information
Budget Planner
CASP critiquing tools
Citethisforme
EndNote
Ginger software
Library search engines
SMART
Spreadsheets
SWOT review

Cardboard, foam logs and pins
Pocket Calculator
Stress ball
Worry stone

BBC Bitesize
Digital recorder
Grammarly
Mindfulness exercises
Progress chart
Reflective journal
Reflective blog
Regional Training Organisations and Network
Training Events Programme
Ongoing Achievement Record
Refme
Research folder
Rewordify
Timetable

Appraisal documents
CPD journal – notebook, 5-year diary, online logbook,
electronic/written portfolio
Diary
Index cards
Journal
NMC Training Toolkit
Nursing Portal
Positive slogan cards
Practice Placement Competency Booklet
Your learning portfolio

APPENDIX 1
LEGISLATIVE POLICIES

University Student Charter

NMC Practice Placement Charter

Adults with Incapacity (Scotland) Act (2000)

Children and Young People (Scotland) Act (2014)

Department of Health, Social Services and Public Safety (2008)

Equality Act (2010)

Health Act (1999)

Health and Social Care Act (2012)

Health Protection Scotland (2015)

Joint Public Bodies Act (2014)

NMC Administration of Medication (2007) regulates your practice based on the UK Medicines Act (1968)

NMC Standards for Pre-registration Midwifery Education (2009)

NMC Standards for Pre-registration Nursing Education (2010)

NMC Midwives Rules and Standards (2012)

NMC Code: Professional Standards of Practice and Behaviour for Nurses and Midwives (2015)

Public Health England (2016)

Public Health Wales (2014)

Safeguarding children and young people – every nurse's responsibility (RCN, 2014)

Safeguarding Vulnerable Groups Act (2006)

The Children Act (2004)

The Mental Health Act (1983, revised 2007)

The Mental Health (Care and Treatment) Act Scotland (2003)

The Mental Health (Amendment, Northern Ireland) Order (2004)

FURTHER READING 📖

www.legislation.gov.uk/

APPENDIX 2
ACTIVITY 1.3 ANSWERS

Visual
Auditory
Auditory
Visual
Tactile
Auditory
Tactile
Visual
Auditory
Tactile
Visual
Tactile

APPENDIX 3
PRACTICE LEARNING PLACEMENTS

ADULT NURSING

Community Health, Primary Care, Secondary Acute Care, Long-term Care, Adult Health setting

CHILD HEALTH

Assessment Unit, Neonatal Intensive Care Unit, Community, Acute Child Health setting, Acute Paediatric Ward, Primary Care, Acute Adult Care, Ambulatory Care, Hospice, Third Sector, Child and Family Centre, Child Development Centre

MENTAL HEALTH

Day Service/Community, Mental Health Care, Continuing Care Elderly/Day Care/Nursing Home, Medical/Surgical, Enduring Mental Health, Acute Mental Health under 65s, Community Mental Health Team, Day Hospital for under 65s, Elderly Acute Assessment, Intensive Psychiatric Care Unit/Crisis out of hours, Complex Mental Health Care, Community Mental Health, Elective Placement

LEARNING DISABILITIES

Residential, Community, 24-hour Care, Nursing Home, Primary Care, Acute and Critical Care, Prison, Forensic Care, Adult, Older Persons and Child and Adolescent Inpatient and Community Mental Health Services, Self-Advocacy Groups, Assessment and Treatment Centre for people with learning disabilities experiencing mental health issues, Day Care

MIDWIFERY

Hospital Maternity Unit, smaller stand-alone Maternity Unit, Private Maternity Hospital, Group Practice, Birth Centre, Community Practice, GP Surgery

APPENDIX 4
PROCRASTINATOR TYPES

Type	Descriptor
Avoider	You believe the task will go away or do itself, so you avoid thinking or doing anything about it.
Browser	Your believable reason for not getting started is that you never feel you've enough information, so you browse the internet, search engines, journals, books, TV documentaries, and still you feel that isn't enough, and so the browsing continues.
Busy-B-er	You busy yourself with lots of other things and nothing much at all justifies your excuse for not doing what actually needs to be done.
Contrary	Your favourite phrase is 'I'll do it when I'm good and ready', but that good and ready time never really comes around and then it's too late.
Deadline-wirer	You feel you work best under pressure and so keep the deadline as your excuse for not getting started, struggling to finish when you're right down to the wire.
Dilly-dally-er	You say you'll get started but you find an excuse for pottering around, doing a bit of this, a bit of that but not what should be getting done.
Dreamer	You constantly dream about being finished but never do anything about getting started so you can get to the finishing point.
Excuse-maker	You keep making excuses for not getting started.
Fail-fearer	You're so scared you aren't up to the mark, of failing and being criticised that you keep putting off getting started, letting anxiety take over.
Guilt-tripper	You feel guilty for putting things off; you try getting started but can't and so get stuck on the guilt trip.

Type	Descriptor
Jumper-hopper	You jump around from one thing to the next, the same-old backwards and forwards, and so hop over and ignore the real task at hand.
Lazy	You can't be bothered even thinking about the task, never mind doing anything to get started.
Over-doer	You gather too much information, take on too much and then can't see the wood for the trees.
Over-loader	You've difficulty saying 'no' and so take on too much and then feel overwhelmed with tasks.
Perfectionist	You never seem happy with what you've produced, going over and over things, hoping to make it all perfect.
Pessimist	You're so afraid of getting it wrong and failing that you believe this will actually happen.
Pile-it-on-er	You've an 'I can manage' attitude and so are happy to take on more and more 'avoidance' jobs; a prime excuse for not getting on with the things you should.
Pottering-jotter	You jot this and that down to do it later, but you just carry on pottering around doing the wrong 'this and that'.
Putter-offer	You do any other mundane task rather than what you actually should be doing.
Stresser	You use up so much energy stressing about the task that you find it hard to focus and get going.
Unmotivated	You can't be bothered; you're not at all interested at the moment.
Worrier	You constantly fret about not managing and failing.

(adapted from Gribben 2012)

APPENDIX 5
ACCESSIBLE POWERPOINTS – WHAT WORKS; WHAT DOESN'T

What works	What doesn't
Dark background with light text for a dark room and the reverse for a well-lit room	Dark print on dark background
No more than two colours of font, e.g. black and blue	Lots of colour; red or green text
Sans serif font – Arial or Verdana	Mix and match too many fonts or use a serif font
28- or 32-point font for PowerPoint; 30–40-point font for OHP	Anything less than a 12-point font for handouts
Left aligned, unjustified text	Justified text; centred text
Double spacing (or 1.5 minimum)	Single spacing
Mix of upper and lower case	ALL CAPITALS
Use of boxes to emphasise or highlight important text	**Bold**, <u>underline</u>, *italics*
Maximum of six bullet points or numbers	One graphical detail dissolving into the next
Presentation of text and pictures separately	Overlapping text and pictures
Horizontal, unangled, text, pictures or diagrams	Angled, moving or horizontal and vertical combination of text, pictures or diagrams
Clear, visible text on diagrams, graphs or tables	Overuse of animation
Use of visuals instead of text where possible	Floating or moving text

APPENDIX 6
REFLECTIVE MODELS

JOHNS' MODEL OF REFLECTION

Describe	The situation and what happened.
Reflect	What you experienced and how you feel.
Influencing factors	Your actions; others' actions and consequences.
Done differently	Alternative actions, approach and consequences
Learning	Enhanced your understanding; altered your approach

(adapted from Johns 2002)

APPENDIX 7
CAREERS INFORMATION

All Cruise Jobs: www.allcruisejobs.com/
Australian Nursing and Midwifery Accreditation Council:
www.anmac.org.au/
Best Job Interview: www.best-job-interview.com/
BMI Healthcare Jobs: https://bmihealthcarejobs.co.uk/
BUPA Careers: www.bupa.co.uk/
Cruise ship medical jobs: www.cruiseshipjob.com/
Goinglobal: www.goinglobal.com/
Health Jobs UK: https://healthjobsuk.com/
Health Professionals Ministry of Health Singapore:
www.moh.gov.sg/content/moh_web/healthprofessionalsportal/all
healthcareprofessionals.html
Health and Social Care Jobs in Northern Ireland: www.hscrecruit.com/
Irish Nursing Board: www.nmbi.ie/
Jobs4Medical: www.jobs4medical.co.uk/
JustforNurses: www.justfornurses.co.uk/
NHS Careers: www.healthcareers.nhs.uk
NHS Jobs (England and Wales): www.jobs.nhs.uk/
NHS Jobs Scotland: https://jobs.scot.nhs.uk/
Nuffield Health Careers: www.nuffieldhealthcareers.com/
Nurses: www.nurses.co.uk/
Nursing and Midwifery Council – Working Outside the UK:
www.nmc.org.uk/registration/working-outside-the-uk/
Nursing Council of New Zealand: www.nursingcouncil.org.nz/
NursingNetUK: nursingnetuk.com/
Nursing Times Jobs: www.nursingtimesjobs.com/
Prospects: www.prospects.ac.uk/

Queen Alexandra's Royal Army Nursing Corps: http://qaranc.co.uk/

RCM: www.rcm.org.uk/

RCN: https://careers.rcn.org.uk/

Redgoldfish: www.redgoldfish.co.uk/

Royal Air Force jobs: www.raf.mod.uk/recruitment/roles/roles-finder? category=medical-and-medical-support

Royal Navy: www.royalnavy.mod.uk/careers

Singapore Nursing Board: www.healthprofessionals.gov.sg/content/hprof/snb/en.html

Skills for Health: www.skillsforhealth.org.uk/

South African Nursing Council: www.sanc.co.za/

Spire Healthcare: www.spirehealthcare.com/

Staff Nurse: www.staffnurse.com/

TARGETjobs: https://targetjobs.co.uk/

Wikijob: www.wikijob.co.uk/

APPENDIX 8
NURSING JOBS

ADULT NURSING

Acute services (medical, surgical, accident and emergency)
Continuing care for the elderly
Specialist roles (e.g. diabetes, multiple sclerosis, epilepsy)
Prison services
Intermediate care (outreach nurse, district nurse, health visitor)
Health promotion (e.g. smoking, sexual health)
Community roles (General Practitioner surgeries, school nurse, family planning, occupational health, NHS Direct/Walk-in Centres)

CHILD HEALTH NURSING

Acute settings (accident and emergency, specialist or generic inpatient wards (specialist or generic), day care and assessment clinics)
Community settings (generic services, specialist roles, e.g. cystic fibrosis, cancer, palliative care)
Specialist roles (e.g. renal, burns and plastics, pain management, complementary medicine)

LEARNING DISABILITIES NURSING

Support accommodation
Hospital settings
Secure environments

Specialist roles, e.g. autism
Health promotion e.g. Wellwoman, Wellmen schemes

MENTAL HEALTH NURSING

Community roles
Educational institutions
Assertive outreach
Rehabilitation
Forensic services
Prison services
Therapist roles
Substance misuse
Child protection
Adolescence services
Specialist roles, e.g. schizophrenia, eating disorders

MIDWIFERY

Hospital (maternity units in general hospital, small stand-alone units, private maternity)
Birth centres
General Practitioner surgeries
Community healthcare settings
Educational institutions
(see www.prospects.ac.uk/job-profiles)

APPENDIX 9
PROFESSIONAL LINKS

GENERAL INFORMATION

www.england.nhs.uk/ourwork/part-rel/scn/
www.nursing-portal.com/index.asp

APPRAISALS

www.nhsemployers.org/your-workforce/retain-and-improve/man
aging-your-workforce/appraisals/appraisal-tools-and-tips

CPD TRAINING FOR NURSES AND MIDWIVES

www.bda.uk.com/professional/cpd1/cpdjointstatement
www.britishpainsociety.org/static/uploads/resources/files/RCN_
KSF_2015.pdf
www.cec.hscni.net/
www.flyingstart.scot.nhs.uk/learning-programmes/cpd/regulation-
and-cpd/
Health Careers, Training and Development (Adult Nursing):
www.healthcareers.nhs.uk/explore-roles/nursing/adult-nurse/t
raining-and-development-adult-nursing
Health Careers, Training and Development (Midwifery): www.health
careers.nhs.uk/explore-roles/midwifery/midwife/training-and-
development-midwifery
www.hee.nhs.uk/hee-your-area
www.hpc-uk.org/registrants/cpd/

learning.wales.nhs.uk/
www.nes.scot.nhs.uk/education-and-training.aspx
www.scottishmaternity.org/

REVALIDATION

Health Careers, Competency Frameworks: www.healthcareers.
nhs.uk/career-planning/developing-your-career/competency-
frameworks
www.nhsemployers.org/SimplifiedKSF
www.nhsemployers.org/your-workforce/retain-and-improve/
standards-and-assurance/professional-regulation/nursing-revalidation
www.nmc.org.uk/globalassets/sitedocuments/revalidation/
how-to-revalidate-booklet.pdf

JOINING A TRADE UNION

my.rcn.org.uk/joining
www.rcm.org.uk/join
www.unison.org.uk/at-work/health-care/representing-you/nursing/
www.unison.org.uk/join/

APPENDIX 10
SMART

You want to find out more about water births, and wonder if there are any courses or if you'd be able to spend time in the regional delivery unit. So, be SMART:

S = Specific (e.g. I want to be able to supervise a water birth alone)

M = Measurable (e.g. I want to know when I will be ready to do that)

A = Action-focused (e.g. Today I'll identify a course on this year's regional training programme)

R = Realistic (e.g. I will discuss with my training mentor/the senior midwife how this can fit into my training plan and work schedule)

T = Time-bound (e.g. I will raise the issue with her at our regular one-to-one meeting next week)

REFERENCES

Ackerman, D. and Gross, B.L. (2005) 'My instructor made me do it: task characteristics of procrastination', *Journal of Marketing Education*, 27(1): 5–13.

Adults with Incapacity (Scotland) Act 2000.

All cruise jobs: www.allcruisejobs.com/

Andre, K. and Heartfield, M. (2011) *Nursing and Midwifery Portfolios: Evidence of Continuing Competence*, 2nd edition. Australia: Churchill Livingstone.

APA referencing: www.ukessays.com

Arthur, K. (2012) *Mind Maps: Improve Memory, Concentration, Communication, Organization, Creativity, and Time Management.* New York: Book Stream Publishing Inc.

Australian Nursing & Midwifery Accreditation Council: www.anmac.org.au/

Bach, S. and Grant, A. (2011) *Communication and Interpersonal Skills in Nursing.* Exeter: Learning Matters Ltd.

Barksby, J. (2014) 'Service users' perceptions of student nurses', *Nursing Times*, 111(19): 23–25.

Bassot, B. (2013) *The Reflective Journal.* Hampshire: Palgrave Macmillan.

Baxter Pharmacy Services (2014) *Good Practice for Drug Calculations: A Step-by-step Guide for Nurses, Doctors and All Other Healthcare Professionals.* Berkshire: Baxter Healthcare Ltd.

Beauchamp, T.L. and Childress, J.F. (2013) *Principles of Biomedical Ethics*, 7th edition. Oxford: Oxford University Press.

Best-job-interview.com: www.best-job-interview.com/

Bitesize: www.bbc.co.uk/education

BMI healthcare jobs: https://bmihealthcarejobs.co.uk/

Borrego, M. and Bird, J. (2010) *Careers Uncovered: Nursing and Midwifery.* Surrey: Trotman Publishing.

Breathing space: http://breathingspace.scot/

Brooker, C. and Waugh, A. (eds) (2013) *Foundations of Nursing Practice: Fundamentals of Holistic Care*, 2nd edition. Edinburgh: Mosby Elsevier.

Bryar, R. and Sinclair, M. (eds) (2011) *Theory for Midwifery Practice*, 2nd edition. Hampshire: Palgrave Macmillan.

bubbl.us: https://bubbl.us/

Bulman, C. and Schutz, S. (eds) (2013) *Reflective Practice in Nursing*, 5th edition. Chichester: John Wiley & Sons Ltd.

BUPA: www.bupa.co.uk/

Byrom, S. and Downe, S. (eds) (2015) *The Roar Behind the Silence: Why Kindness, Compassion and Respect Matter in Maternity Care.* London: Pinter and Martin Ltd.

Cabellero, C., Creed, F., Gochmanski, C. and Lovegrove, J. (2012) *Nursing OSCEs: A Complete Guide to Exam Success.* Oxford: Oxford University Press.

The Cambridge Student (2016) 'Procrastination: peril of the perfectionist', www.tcs.cam.ac.uk/features/0033285-procrastination-peril-of-the-perfectionist.html

Care Inspectorate (2016) 'About us': www.careinspectorate.com/index.php/about-us

Care Quality Commission (CQC) (2016) 'Who we are': www.cqc.org.uk/content/who-we-are

CASP: www.casp-uk.net/#!untitled/checklists/cb36

CETL learning: www.cetl.org.uk/learning/

The Children Act 2004.

Children and Young People (Scotland) Act 2014

Citethisforme.com: www.citethisforme.com/

Claro software: www.clarosoftware.com/

Clinical Education Centre: www.cec.hscni.net/

Cluett, E. and Bluff, R.E. (2006) *Principles and Practice of Research in Midwifery.* Philadelphia: Elsevier.

Colley, S. (2003) 'Nursing theory: its importance to practice', *Nursing Standard,* 17(46): 33–37.

Concept Northern: www.conceptnorthern.co.uk

Coombs, J. (2015) *Nurses Reflective Diary: Revalidation.* Colorado Springs: CreateSpace Independent Publishing Platform.

Cruise Ship Jobs: www.cruiseshipjob.com/

CSSIW (2016) 'Our reports': http://cssiw.org.uk/our-reports/?lang=en

Davey, L. and Houghton, D. (2013) *The Midwife's Pocket Formulary,* 3rd edition. London: Churchill Livingstone.

Davies, P. (2013) *How To Get Through Revalidation: Making the Process Easy.* Boca Raton FL: CRC Press.

Department of Health (2008, revised 2015) *The Health and Social Care Act 2008: Code of Practice on the Prevention and Control of Infections and Related Guidance.* London: DH.

Department of Health (2009) *Preceptorship Framework for Newly Registered Nurses, Midwives and Allied Health Professionals.* London: DH.

Department of Health and Public Health England (2013) *The Evidence Base of the Public Health Contribution of Nurses and Midwives.* London: DH and Public Health England.

Department of Health: Chief Nursing Officers of England, Northern Ireland, Scotland and Wales (2010) Midwifery 2020: Delivering Expectations. London: Department of Health (www.gov.uk/government/uploads/system/uploads/attachment_data/file/216029/dh_119470.pdf

Department of Health, Social Services and Public Safety (2011) *The Northern Ireland Regional Infection Prevention and Control Manual Infection Control Guidelines*. Northern Ireland: DHSSPS.

Duffy, K. (2013) 'Providing constructive feedback to students during mentoring', *Nursing Standard*, 27(31): 50–56.

Egan, G. (2013) *The Skilled Helper: A Problem-Management and Opportunity Development Approach to Helping*, 10th edition. Belmont: Brooks/Cole.

El-Gilany, A.H. and Abusaad, F.E.S. (2012) 'Self-directed learning readiness and learning styles among Saudi undergraduate nursing students', *Nurse Education Today*, 33(9): 1040–1044.

Endnote: http://endnote.com/

England, C. and Morgan, R. (2012) *Communication Skills for Midwives: Challenges in Everyday Practice*. Maidenhead: Open University Press.

Equality Act (2010)

Evidence-Based Nursing: http://ebn.bmj.com/site/podcasts/

Facebook: www.facebook.com/

Fearon, C. and Nicol, M. (2011) 'Strategies to assist prevention of burnout in nursing staff', *Nursing Standard*, 26(14): 35–39.

Find midwives jobs - https://jobs.midwives.org.uk

Flying Start NHS, Continuing Professional Development: www.flyingstart.scot.nhs.uk/learning-programmes/cpd/regulation-and-cpd/

Flying Start NHS, Research and Evidence Based Practice: Everyone's Responsibility: www.flyingstart.scot.nhs.uk/learning-programmes/research-for-practice/research-and-evidence-based-practice-everyones-responsibility/

Frixione, N., Hettena, J. and Barnes, T. (2015) 'Strategies for coping with the emotional burden in nursing': https://prezi.com/ltyveq5uvnnz/strategies-for-coping-with-the-emotional-burden-in-nursing/

Galanti, G.A. (2008) *Caring for Patients from Different Cultures*, 4th edition. Pennsylvania: University of Pennsylvania Press.

Garrison, K. and Lacey, A. (eds) (2015) *The Research Process in Nursing*, 7th edition. West Sussex: Wiley-Blackwell.

General Medical Council, Members' Code of Conduct: www.gmc-uk.org/about/council/register_code_of_conduct.asp

George, J. (2010) *Nursing Theories: The Base for Professional Nursing*, 6th edition. Essex: Pearson.

Gibbs, G. (2013) *Learn by Doing: A Guide to Teaching and Learning Methods*. Oxford: FEU.

GINGER: www.gingersoftware.com/

Glassdoor: www.glassdoor.co.uk/index.htm

GMC/NMC (2015) *Openness and Honesty When Things Go Wrong: The Professional Duty of Candour*. London: GMC/NMC.

Going Global: www.goinglobal.com/

Google Scholar: http://scholar.google.co.uk/

Gopee, L.N. (2003) 'The nurse as a lifelong learner: an exploration of nurses' perceptions of lifelong learning within nursing, and of nurses as lifelong learners'.

PhD thesis, University of Warwick, WRAP: Warwick Research Archive Portal (http://wrap.warwick.ac.uk/).

Gradjobs, 'Using the STAR technique to succeed at interviews': www.gradjobs. co.uk/careers-advice/interview-advice/using-the-star-technique-to-succeed-at-interviews

Graduate Recruitment Bureau: www.grb.uk.com/

Grammarly: www.grammarly.com/

Gribben, M. (2012) The Study Skills Toolkit for Students with Dyslexia. London: SAGE Publications.

Gov.uk, Student Finance: www.gov.uk/student-finance

Hall, A. (2005) 'Defining nursing knowledge', Nursing Times, 101(48): 34.

Hamilton, S., Murray, K., Hamilton, S. and Martin, D. (2015) 'A strategy for maintaining student wellbeing', Nursing Times, 111(7): 20–22.

Harvard referencing: https://libweb.anglia.ac.uk/referencing/harvard.htm

Hassed, C. and Chambers, R. (2014) Mindful Learning: Reduce Stress and Improve Brain Performance for Effective Learning. NSW: Exisle Publishing Pty Ltd.

Haugh, B. (2016) 'Becoming a mother and learning to breastfeed: an emergent autoethnography', Journal of Perinatal Education, 25(1): 56–68.

Health Act 1999.

Health and Social Care Act 2012.

Health & Care Professions Council: www.hcpc-uk.co.uk/

Health & Care Professions Council, Standards of Continuing Professional Development: www.hpc-uk.org/aboutregistration/standards/cpd/

Health & Care Professions Council (2015), Continuing Professional Development: www.hpc-uk.org/registrants/cpd/

Health Careers, Competency Frameworks: www.healthcareers.nhs.uk/career-planning/developing-your-career/competency-frameworks

Health Careers, Training and Development (Adult Nursing): www.health careers.nhs.uk/explore-roles/nursing/adult-nurse/training-and-development-adult-nursing

Health Careers, Training and Development (Midwifery): www.healthcareers. nhs.uk/explore-roles/midwifery/midwife/training-and-development-midwifery

Health Education England, HEE in your area: www.hee.nhs.uk/hee-your-area

The Health Foundation (2014): www.health.org.uk/node/229

healthjobsuk.com: http://healthjobsuk.com/

Health Professionals Ministry of Health Singapore: www.moh.gov.sg/content/ moh_web/healthprofessionalsportal/allhealthcareprofessionals.html

Health Protection Scotland (2015) The National Infection Control Manual. Glasgow: NPSNHS.

Health and Social Care Jobs in Northern Ireland: hserecruit.com: www.hse recruit.com/

Hello my name is…: http://hellomynameis.org.uk/

Hendrick, J. (2004) Law and Ethics: Foundations in Nursing and Healthcare. Chapter 1: 'Law and Ethics'. Cheltenham: Nelson Thornes Ltd. pp. 1–22.

Higher Education Authority: www.hea.ie/

HIS (2016) 'About us': www.healthcareimprovementscotland.org/about_us. aspx

Honey, P. and Mumford, A. (2001) *The Learning Styles Questionnaire*. London: Peter Honey Publications.

Howatson-Jones, L. (2016) *Reflective Practice in Nursing*, 3rd edition. London: SAGE Publications.

Hunter, B. and Deery, R. (eds) (2009) *Emotions in Midwifery and Reproduction*. Hampshire: Palgrave Macmillan.

Hunter, B. and Warren, L. (2013) *Investigating Resilience in Midwifery*. Final Report. Cardiff University: Cardiff (http://orca.cf.ac.uk/61594/).

Hutchfield, K. and Standing, M. (2012) *Succeeding in Essays, Exams and OSCEs*. London: SAGE Publications.

Hutton, M. and Gardner, H. (2005) 'Calculation skills', *Paediatric Nursing*, 17(2). Middlesex: RCN Publishing Company.

Iansyst: www.iansyst.co.uk

Inspiration software: www.inspiration.com/

Irish Nursing Board: www.nmbi.ie/

Jobs4medical: www.jobs4medical.co.uk/

Johns, C. (2002) *Guided Reflection: Advancing Practice*. Oxford: Blackwell Science Ltd.

Johns, C. (2013) *Becoming a Reflective Practitioner*, 4th edition. Oxford: John Wiley & Sons Ltd.

Johnson, R. (2010) *Skills for Midwifery Practice*, 3rd edition. London: Churchill Livingstone.

Johnstone, M.J. (2016) *Bioethics: A Nursing Perspective*, 6th edition. NSW Australia: Elsevier.

Joint Public Bodies Act 2014.

Jones, C. and Hayter, M. (2013) 'Editorial: social media use by nurses and midwives: a "recipe for disaster" or a "force for good"?' *Journal of Clinical Nursing*, 22(11–12): 1495–1496.

Journal of Research in Nursing Podcasts: http://jrn.sagepub.com/site/podcast/podcast_dir.xhtml

Just for Nurses: www.justfornurses.co.uk/

Kelly, J. (2007) *Procrastination*. Royal College of Art Graduation Project (https://vimeo.com/9553205).

Kingdon, C., Neilson, J., Singleton, V., Gyte, G., Hart, A., Gabbay, M. and Lavendar, T. (2009) 'Choice and birth method: mixed method study of caesarean delivery for maternal request', *British Journal of Obstetrics and Gynaecology*, 116(7): 886–895.

Kline, R. with Khan, S. (2013) *The Duty of Care of Healthcare Professionals*. Public World: www.publicworld.org/files/Duty_of_care_handbook_April_2013.pdf.

Kollak, I. (2009) *Yoga for Nurses*. New York: Springer Publishing Company.

Landa, J. and Lopez-Safra, E. (2010) 'The impact of emotional intelligence on nursing: an overview', *Psychology*, 1: 50–58.

LanguageLine: www.languageline.com/uk

Lapham, R. (2015) *Drug Calculations for Nurses: A Step-by-step Approach*, 4th edition. Boca Raton FL: CRC Press.

Learning@NHSWales: https://learning.wales.nhs.uk/

Lee, K.G. (2014) 'Group B streptococcal septicemia of the newborn': https://med lineplus.gov/ency/article/001366.htm

Legislation.gov.uk: www.legislation.gov.uk/

Levett-Jones, T. and Bourgeois, S. (2015) *The Clinical Placement: An Essential Guide for Nursing Students*, 3rd edition. London: Churchill Livingstone.

Lillyman, S., Gutteridge, R. and Berridge, P. (2011) 'Using a storyboarding technique in the classroom to address end of life experiences in practice and engage student nurses in deeper reflection', *Nurse Education Practice*, 11(3): 179–186.

McCormack, B. and McCance, T. (2010) *Person-Centred Nursing: Theory and Practice.* West Sussex: Wiley-Blackwell.

Maslin-Prothero, S. (ed.) (2005) *Bailliere's Study Skills for Nurses and Midwives.* London: Bailliere Tindall.

www.Medincle: www.medincle.com/

The Mental Health Act 1983, revised 2007.

The Mental Health (Care and Treatment) Act Scotland 2003.

The Mental Health (Amendment, Northern Ireland) Order 2004.

Mental Health in Manchester, Self-help guides: www.mhim.org.uk/helpguides/

Midirs, Midwifery podcast: www.midirs.org/podcast/midwifery-podcast-new-students/

Ministry of Health Singapore, All Healthcare Professionals: www.moh.gov.sg/content/ moh_web/healthprofessionalsportal/allhealthcareprofessionals.html

Moodle: moodle.org/

Moon, J. (1999) *Reflection in Learning and Professional Development.* London: Kogan Page.

Mosby (2016) *Mosby's Medical Dictionary*, 10th edition. St Louis, Missouri: Elsevier.

National Union of Students: www.nus.org.uk

NHS 24: www.nhs24.com/

NHS Business Services Authority: www.nhsbsa.nhs.uk/

NHS Choices, Student Stress: www.nhs.uk/LiveWell/Studenthealth/Pages/Coping withstress.aspx

NHS Education for Scotland: www.nes.scot.nhs.uk/

NHS Education for Scotland, Education and Training: www.nes.scot.nhs.uk/ education-and-training.aspx

NHS Education for Scotland (2012a) *Breaking the Chain of Infection* (www.nes. scot.nhs.uk/).

NHS Education for Scotland (2012b) *Legal and Ethics Guidance: Advanced Nursing Practice Toolkit* (www.advancedpractice.scot.nhs.uk/legal-and-ethics-guidance.aspx).

NHS Education for Scotland (2016) *Scottish Multi-professional Maternity Development Programme* (www.nes.scot.nhs.uk/).

NHS Employers, Appraisal tools and tips: www.nhsemployers.org/your-workforce/ retain-and-improve/managing-your-workforce/appraisals/appraisal-tools-and-tips

NHS Employers, Revalidation for nurses and midwives: www.nhsemployers.org/ your-workforce/retain-and-improve/standards-and-assurance/professional-regulation/nursing-revalidation

NHS Employers, Simplified Knowledge and Skills Framework (KSF): www. nhsemployers.org/SimplifiedKSF

NHS England, Strategic Clinical Networks: www.england.nhs.uk/ourwork/part-rel/scn/

NHS England (2016) *Care, Compassion, Competence, Communication, Courage, Commitment: Compassion in Practice – One Year On.* Leeds: NHS England/ Nursing Directorate.

NHS jobs: www.jobs.nhs.uk/

NHS Institute for Innovation and Improvement (2008) *SBAR: Situation, Background, Assessment, Recommendation.* Coventry: NHS Institute for Innovation and Improvement.

NHS Scotland, KSF Guidance: www.ksf.scot.nhs.uk/

NHS Scotland, Recruitment: jobs.scot.nhs.uk/

NHS Scotland (2007) *Delivering for Remote and Rural Healthcare: The Final Report of the Remote and Rural Workstream.* Edinburgh: The Scottish Government.

NICE: www.nice.org.uk/

NICE (2014) *Vitamin D: A Systematic Review of Effectiveness and Cost-Effectiveness of Activities to Increase Awareness, Uptake and Provision of Vitamin D Supplements in at Risk Groups* (www.nice.org.uk/guidance/ph56/ evidence/evidence-review-1-431762365).

NICE (2016) *Antenatal Care Guidelines* (www.nice.org.uk/guidance/cg62).

Nursing and Midwifery Board of Ireland: www.nmbi.ie/Home

NMC: www.nmc.org.uk/

NMC, Informing us of cautions and convictions: www.nmc.org.uk/registration/staying-on-the-register/informing-us-of-cautions-and-convictions/

NMC, Introduction to safeguarding for adults: www.nmc.org.uk/standards/safe guarding/introduction-to-safeguarding-for-adults/

NMC, Midwifery regulation: www.nmc.org.uk/standards/what-to-expect-from-a-nurse-or-midwife/midwifery/midwifery-regulation/

NMC, Revalidation: revalidation.nmc.org.uk/

NMC (2009) *Standards for Pre-registration Midwifery Education.* London: NMC.

NMC (2010) *Standards for Pre-registration Nursing Education.* London: NMC.

NMC (2012) *Rules and Standards for Midwives.* London: NMC.

NMC (2014) *Standards for Competence for Registered Nurses.* London: NMC.

NMC (2015a) *The Code: Professional Standards of Practice and Behaviour for Nurses and Midwives.* London: NMC (www.nmc.org.uk/standards/code).

NMC (2015b) *Raising Concerns: Guidance for Nurses and Midwives.* London: NMC (www.nmc.org.uk/standards/guidance/raising-concerns-guidance-for-nurses-and-midwives/).

NMC (2015c) *How to Revalidate with the NMC: Requirements for Renewing your Registration.* London: NMC (www.nmc.org.uk/globalassets/sitedocuments/ revalidation/how-to-revalidate-booklet.pdf).

NMC (2016) *Social Media Guidance*. London: NMC.

NPSA (2004) *Seven Steps to Patient Safety: An Overview Guide for NHS Staff*. London: NHS (www.nrls.npsa.nhs.uk/resources/collections/seven-steps-to-patient-safety/).

Nuffield Health, Careers: www.nuffieldhealthcareers.com/

Nurses.co.uk: www.nurses.co.uk/

Nursing Careers: http://nursing.nhscareers.nhs.uk/careers

Nursing Council of New Zealand: www.nursingcouncil.org.nz/

Nursingnetuk.com: www.nursingnetuk.com/

The Nursing Portal: www.nursing-portal.com/index.asp

Nursing Standard, 'Art of good communication': http://journals.rcni.com/page/ns/students/clinical-placements/patientcentred-care/art-of-good-communication

Nursing Times, jobs.com: www.nursingtimesjobs.com/

Open Athens: www.openathens.net/

O'Shea, E. (2003) 'Self-directed learning in nursing education: a review of the literature', *Journal of Advanced Nursing*, 43(1): 62–70.

Osman, S.E., Tischler, V. and Schneider, J. (2014) '"Singing for the brain": a qualitative study exploring the health and well-being benefits of singing for people with dementia and their carers', *Dementia*, published online, 24 November.

Owen, R. and Candelier, C.K. (2010) 'A "modified" CHAPs tool – an effective system for handover of care between medical staff in a maternity unit setting', *Archives of Disease in Childhood: Fetal and Neonatal Edition*, 95: 66–67.

Oxford Dictionaries (2013) *Primary Maths: Oxford Primary Illustrated Maths Dictionary*. Oxford: Oxford University Press.

Parahoo, K. (2014) *Nursing Research Principles, Process and Issues*. Basingstoke: Palgrave Macmillan.

Pavord, E. and Donnelly, E. (2015) *Communication and Interpersonal Skills*, 2nd edition. Banbury: Lantern Publishing.

Penumbra: www.penumbra.org.uk/

Peplau, H.E. (1991) *Interpersonal Relations in Nursing: A Conceptual Framework of Reference for Psychodynamic Nursing*. New York: Springer Publishing Co. Inc.

Perry, A. (2003) *The Little Book of Procrastination: How to Stop Putting Things Off*. Suffolk: Worth Publishing Ltd.

Plagiarism.org: www.plagiarism.org/

Polit, D. and Beck, C. (2014) *Essentials of Nursing Research Appraising Evidence for Nursing Practice*. Philadelphia: Lippincott, Williams and Wilkins.

Price, B. and Harrington, A. (2016) *Critical Thinking and Writing Skills for Nursing Students*, 3rd edition. London: SAGE Publications.

Prospects: www.prospects.ac.uk/

Public Health Wales (2014) *National Infection Control Policies for Wales* (www.wales.nhs.uk/).

Pychyl, T.A. (2013) *Solving the Procrastination Puzzle: A Concise Guide to Strategies for Change*. New York: Penguin.

QARANC – Queen Alexandra's Royal Army Nursing Corps: http://qaranc.co.uk/

Royal Air Force, Roles finder: www.raf.mod.uk/recruitment/roles/roles-finder? category=medical-and-medical-support

RCM: www.rcm.org.uk/

RCM, Join: www.rcm.org.uk/join

RCN: www.rcn.org.uk/

RCN, Careers: careers.rcn.org.uk

RCN, Join the Royal College of Nursing: www.rcn.org.uk/join; https://my.rcn.org. uk/joining

RCN Joint Position Statement: www.bda.uk.com/professional/cpd1/cpdjoint statement

Redgoldfish.co.uk: www.redgoldfish.co.uk/

Redgoldfish.co.uk, Cruise ship jobs: www.redgoldfish.co.uk/cruise-ships-jobs

Rees, C. (2011) *Introduction to Research for Midwives*, 3rd edition. Edinburgh: Churchill Livingstone/Elsevier.

Referencing Made Easy: www.refme.com/

The Regulation and Quality Improvement Authority (RQIA) (2016) Who we are: www.rqia.org.uk

Reid, B. (1993) 'But we're doing it already! Exploring a response to the concept of reflective practice in order to improve its facilitation', *Nurse Education Today*, 13(4): 305–309.

Rewordify.com: https://rewordify.com/

RNAO, Careers in nursing: http://careersinnursing.ca/new-grads-and-job-seekers/ career-services/career-mapping

Robertson, J., Roberts, H., Emerson, E., Turner, S. and Greig, R. (2010) *Health Checks for People with Learning Disabilities: A Systematic Review of Evidence*. London: Improving Health and Lives; Learning Disabilities Observatory.

Roche, M. (2013) *The Sketchmore Handbook: The Illustrated Guide to Visual Note-taking*. Berkeley, CA: Peachpit Press.

Rolfe, G., Freshwater, D. and Jasper, M. (2001) *Critical Reflection in Nursing and the Helping Professions: A User's Guide*. Basingstoke: Palgrave Macmillan.

Royal College of Midwifery: www.rcm.org.uk/

Royal College of Nursing (RCN) (2005) *Good Practice in Infection Prevention and Control: Guidance for Nursing Staff*. London: RCN.

Royal College of Nursing (RCN) (2009) *Integrated Core Career and Competence Framework for Registered Nurses*. London: RCN.

Royal College of Nursing (RCN) (2014a) *Safeguarding Children and Young People: Every Nurse's Responsibility*. London: RCN.

Royal College of Nursing (RCN) (2014b) *Infection and Prevention Control: Information and Learning Resources for Healthcare Staff*. London: RCN.

Royal College of Nursing (RCN) (2015a) *RCN Mentorship Project 2015: From Today's Support in Practice to Tomorrow's Vision for Excellence*. London: RCN.

Royal College of Nursing (RCN) (2015b) *Accountability and Delegation: Information on Accountability and Delegation for all Members of the Nursing Team*. London: RCN.

Royal College of Nursing (RCN) (2015c) *Safeguarding Adults – Everyone's Responsibility. RCN Guidance for Nursing Staff*. London: RCN.

Royal College of Nursing (RCN) (2015d) *RCN Pain Knowledge and Skills Framework for the Nursing Team*. London: RCN (www.britishpainsociety.org/static/uploads/resources/files/RCN_KSF_2015.pdf).

Royal Navy, Careers: www.royalnavy.mod.uk/careers

Safeguarding Vulnerable Groups Act 2006.

Saks, M. and Allsop, J. (2012) *Researching Health: Qualitative, Quantitative and Mixed Methods*, 2nd edition. London: SAGE Publications.

Samaritans: www.samaritans.org/

SANE: www.sane.org.uk/

Schneider, Z., Whitehead, D., LoBiondo-Wood, G. and Haber, J. (2012) *Nursing and Midwifery Research: Methods and Appraisal for Evidence-based Practice*, 4th edition. London: Mosby.

Schön, D. (1983) The Reflective Practitioner. Aldershot: Avebury. In Johns, C. (2013) *Becoming a Reflective Practitioner*, 4th edition. Oxford: John Wiley & Sons Ltd.

Schön, D. (1987) Educating the Reflective Practitioner. San Francisco, CA: Jossey-Bass. In Johns, C. (2013) *Becoming a Reflective Practitioner*, 4th edition. Oxford: John Wiley & Sons Ltd.

Scottish Maternity: www.scottishmaternity.org/

Scovell, S. (2010) 'Role of the nurse-to-nurse handover in patient care', *Nursing Standard*, 24(20): 35–39.

Scrivener, R., Hand, T. and Hooper, R. (2011) 'Accountability and responsibility: principle of nursing practice B', *Nursing Standard*, 25(29): 35–36.

seAp (2015) Advocacy Code of Practice: www.seap.org.uk/

Shifthub: http://shifthub.com/

Shorter, M. and Stayt, L. (2010) 'Critical care nurses' experiences of grief in an adult intensive care unit', *Journal of Advanced Nursing*, 66(1): 159–167.

SIGN: www.sign.ac.uk/

Singapore Nursing Board: www.healthprofessionals.gov.sg/content/hprof/snb/en.html

Skills for Health: www.skillsforhealth.org.uk/

Skills You Need, Reflective Practice: www.skillsyouneed.com/ps/reflective-practice.html

Smoker, A. (2016) *Launching Your Career in Nursing and Midwifery: A Practical Guide*. London: Palgrave.

Snapchat: www.snapchat.com/

Somerville, D. and Keeling, J. (2004) 'A practical approach to promote reflective practice within nursing', *Nursing Times*, 100(12): 42–45.

South African Nursing Council: www.sanc.co.za/

Spire Healthcare: www.spirehealthcare.com/

Staffnurse.com: www.staffnurse.com/

Steel, P. (2011) *The Procrastination Equation: How to Stop Putting Things Off and Start Getting Stuff Done*. Harlow: Pearson Education Limited.

Stone, J. (2011) *Minding the Bedside: Nursing from the Heart of the Awakened Mind*. Minneapolis: Langdon Street Press.

Student Awards Agency Scotland: www.saas.gov.uk/

Student Finance: www.gov.uk/student-finance/

Student Finance England: www.sfengland.slc.co.uk/

Student Finance NI: www.studentfinanceni.co.uk

Student Finance Wales: www.studentfinancewales.co.uk/

The Student Room, 'How to cope on nursing placements': www.thestudentroom.co.uk/wiki/how_to_cope_on_nursing_placements

Studymore.org.uk, 'Time management tips from students': www.studymore.org.uk/timetips.htm

Sully, P. and Dallas, J. (2010) *Essential Communication Skills for Nursing and Midwifery (Essential Skills for Nurses)*. Edinburgh: Mosby.

Targetjobs: https://targetjobs.co.uk/

Taylor, B.J. (2006) *Reflective Practice: A Guide for Nurses and Midwives*, 2nd edition. Glasgow: Open University Press.

Taylor, D.B. (2012) *Writing Skills for Nursing and Midwifery Students*. London: SAGE Publications.

Tefula, M. (2014) *Student Procrastination: Seize the Day and Get More Work Done*. Hampshire: Palgrave Macmillan.

Testandcalc: www.testandcalc.com/

Tett, L., Hounsell, J., Cree, V., Christie, H. and McCune, V. (2012) 'Learning from feedback? Mature students' experiences of assessment of higher education', *Research of Post-Compulsory Education*, 17(2): 247–260.

Thompson, S. and Thompson, N. (2008) *The Critically Reflective Practitioner*. Hampshire: Palgrave Macmillan.

Thurston, C. (ed.) (2013) *Essential Nursing Care for Children and Young People: Theory, Policy and Practice*. Abingdon, Oxon: Routledge.

Turnitin: www.turnitinuk.com/

Twitter: https://twitter.com/

UK Essays, Annotated bibliography: www.ukessays.com/essays/health/annotated-bibliography.php

UNISON: www.unison.org.uk/

The University of Manchester Counselling Service (2016): www.counsellingservice.manchester.ac.uk/procrastination/

VAK Learning Styles Self-Assessment Questionnaire: www.businessballs.com/freepdfmaterials/vak_learning_styles_questionnaire.pdf

VARK: http://vark-learn.com/

http://vark-learn.com/the-vark-questionnaire/

Video scribe: www.videoscribe.co/

Weimer, M. (2013) *Learner-Centered Teaching: Five Key Changes to Practice*, 2nd edition. San Francisco, CA: Jossey-Bass.

Whitehead, B. (2013) 'Getting the most out of your clinical placement', *Nursing Times*, 109(37): 12–13.

Whitehead, E. and Mason, T. (2003) *Study Skills for Nurses*. London: SAGE Publications.

WHO, Infection control standard precautions in health care: www.who.int/csr/resources/publications/4EPR_AM2.pdf

WHO (2006) *Infection Control Standard Precautions in Health Care*. Geneva: World Health Organization.

WHO (2011) *Strengthening Midwifery Toolkit: Competencies for Midwifery Practice Module 4*. Geneva: World Health Organization.

WikiJob: www.wikijob.co.uk/

Wise mapping: www.wisemapping.com/

Zen Habits, 'Breaking the fears that cause procrastination': http://zenhabits.net/procrastination-fears/

INDEX